VOID
Library of Davidson College

Worldwatch Paper 59

Improving World Health:
A Least Cost Strategy

William U. Chandler

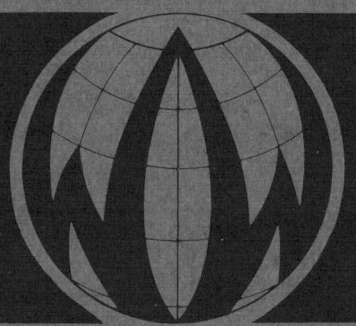

July 1984

Worldwatch Institute is an independent, nonprofit research organization created to analyze and to focus attention on global problems. Directed by Lester R. Brown, Worldwatch is funded by private foundations and United Nations organizations. Worldwatch papers are written for a worldwide audience of decision makers, scholars, and the general public.

Improving World Health:
A Least Cost Strategy

William U. Chandler

Worldwatch Paper 59
July 1984

350.77
C456 i

Sections of this paper may be reproduced in magazines and newspapers with acknowledgment to Worldwatch Institute. The views expressed are those of the author and do not necessarily represent those of Worldwatch Institute and its directors, officers, or staff.

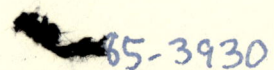
85-3930

©Copyright Worldwatch Institute, 1984
Library of Congress Catalog Card Number 84-51598
ISBN 0-916468-59-3

Printed on recycled paper

Table of Contents

Introduction 5

Primary Health Care 8

Drinking Water and Toilets 20

Low-risk Diets 29

Anti-smoking Measures 39

High Technology 45

Conclusion 51

Notes 55

Introduction

World health leaders have set a goal of "health for all by the year 2000," a step that has initiated a global effort to define health and to devise ways to achieve it.[1] One natural place to begin is with the world's principal causes of death. A large number of early deaths are preventable, and many more lives can be extended into old age. These lives can be saved for a surprisingly low cost.

Death, as characterized by Euripides in his tragedy *Alcestis*, said, "Those who could afford a late death would buy it." Nations that could afford it have invested heavily in medicine and sanitation, and as a result, their children are ten times more likely to survive to adulthood than the children of the least affluent.[2] Adults in richer lands also live longer, although, ironically, many now die prematurely of diseases associated with affluence.

Though their health care needs differ drastically, the rich and the poor do have one thing in common: both die unnecessarily. The rich die of heart disease and cancer, the poor die of diarrhea, pneumonia, and measles. (See Table 1.) Scientific medicine could vastly reduce the mortality caused by these illnesses. Yet, half the developing world lacks medical care of any kind.[3] The rich, though infinitely better cared for, have had to begin rationing health care in the face of rising costs. A policy of health for all can succeed, therefore, only if limited resources are used in the most efficient way possible.

Death is inevitable, of course, but its occurence in either infancy or middle age has importance beyond the obvious meaning for the individual. High infant mortality rates portend a generation with reduced capacity for learning and work—for human development. Reduced mortality rates indicate a general improvement in health.

I would like to thank Brian Brown and Susan Norris for assistance in the preparation of this paper, and George Alleyne, David Banta, Clyde Behney, Peter Bourne, John Foggle, Hellen Gelband, Davidson Gwatkin, Holly Gwin, James Heiby, Judith Jacobsen, Michael Jacobson, and Larry Miike for reviewing the manuscript.

Table 1: Causes of Death In Rich and Poor Countries, 1980

Disease or Cause of Death	Developed Countries[1]	Developing Countries[2]
	(percent)	
Diarrheal Infections and Parasites	1	17
Respiratory Infections	8	18
Heart Disease and Strokes	48	18
Cancer	21	8
Accidents	7	7
Other	15	32
Total	100	100

[1] Seventy-five percent of all developed countries. [2] Chile, Peru, Mexico, Iran, and Philippines, unweighted average.

Source: World Health Organization Data Bank.

Likewise, reducing catastrophic heart attack in middle age not only prolongs and improves the lives of individuals, but saves for society its most productive members.

Impressive improvements in human health have been made recently in rich and poor countries alike. Since 1960, average life expectancy in 34 of the world's poorest countries has increased from 41 to 50 years. Much of this improvement is due to reduced infant mortality, brought about by adoption of modern medicine and improving economic conditions. With the worldwide economic recession, these improvements have slowed somewhat.

In developed nations, life expectancy was increased from an average of 70 to more than 75 years.[4] Several countries, including the United States, France, and the Netherlands, now spend over 8 percent of their entire economic output on health care. Developed nations, in fact, now spend more money on health care than the poorest half of

> "Developed nations now spend more money on health care than the poorest half of the world spends on all items."

the world spends on all items. The poor countries, many of which already allot half of their health care budgets to hospital-based care that reaches only a few, cannot hope to provide high levels of care in the near future. Waiting for incomes to rise will work far too slowly to help the present generation, because half the world cannot reasonably expect to earn more than $1,500 per capita by the year 2010.[5] At the same time, China, Costa Rica, Cuba, Chile, Sri Lanka and others have shown that major improvements in health can be accomplished at low income levels. Statistical analysis shows a low correlation between rates of infant death and income levels up to $2,000 per capita.[6]

Fortunately, major improvements in world health can be made with cost-effective preventive and primary care measures. The most important of these are providing maternal and child care for the world's poorest people, clean drinking water and sanitation facilities to the third of the world's population that lacks them, diet education for populations at high risk of heart disease and cancer, control of tobacco products, and basic research for low-cost cures.[7]

But the largest opportunities for reducing unnecessary death today go untaken. In developing countries, simple diarrhea will kill more people this decade than the Bubonic Plague throughout the Middle Ages.[8] Pneumonia will take a comparable toll. Most of the victims of these diseases will be young children. In India, Kenya, and Guatemala, for example, half of all deaths occur in children under five years of age. Respiratory and diarrheal diseases account for more than two-thirds of all childhood deaths in many developing countries. For those who survive childhood, life spans average six to eight years less than in developed countries; one month in ten is seriously disrupted by sickness. Trachoma, preventable with hygiene and curable with inexpensive antibiotics, has blinded 2 million people. Sleeping sickness retards rural economic development in a wide area of Africa by killing both animals and humans. Malaria kills people or deprives them of the energy for work throughout Africa, Asia, and South America. The list of other tropical ailments is long.[9]

When children die in the developed lands, it usually is in an automobile accident, fire, or fall. Measles, whooping cough, and diphtheria have been virtually eliminated as causes of death. Birth defects still take their toll, but even so, only 3 percent of all infant and child deaths occur in the developed world.[10] Many adults in industrialized countries, however, die prematurely as a result of avoidable effects of heart disease and cancer. About 40 percent of all cancer and 25 percent of all heart disease deaths in the United States, for example, occur in persons younger than sixty-five.[11] Although these degenerative diseases may be inevitable in late old age, perhaps half of the deaths in persons younger than sixty-five could be avoided with preventive medicine. The quality of life for many others could be vastly improved.[12]

Many people still do not understand the health risks they face. Sudanese women, for example, believe that during pregnancy it is harmful to their unborn children to eat eggs or fish, their major sources of protein. This attitude accounts in part for the low birth weights and high infant mortality in that part of Africa.[13] Similarly, many Americans do not yet understand the role of cholesterol and fat in producing heart disease and cancer. Most people in developed countries, in fact, have been taught that dairy products and meat are nearly perfect foods, and that eating more protein and less carbohydrates is good for them. Both groups can benefit most from that basic function of public health care, teaching people to help themselves. As David Banta of the Pan American Health Organization advises, "Never begin with the premise that people will not act on information."[14]

Primary Health Care

Lowering infant and child mortality in developing lands offers the greatest opportunity in the world today for saving lives at a low cost. One-quarter of all deaths, totaling 15 million per year, occur among children under the age of five, and of these, two-thirds are infants, that is, less than a year old. Ninety-seven percent of these deaths befall developing countries, primarily nations where population growth is rapid. Three million infants die annually in India alone. Infant deaths in Bangladesh, Nigeria, Indonesia, and Pakistan together total some two million each year.[15]

> "Ninety-seven percent of infant deaths befall developing countries."

Children of the Third World die of diseases usually not considered lethal elsewhere. Diarrhea, complicated or brought on by malnutrition, causes about a third of all child and infant deaths. Pneumonia vies with diarrheal diseases as the leading taker of young life. Measles, one of the most infectious diseases known, makes children more susceptible to pneumonia, though it is preventable by vaccination. Tetanus, whooping cough, diphtheria, and tuberculosis, also preventable by vaccinations, continue to take a heavy toll.[16]

Comparison with the developed world indicates the magnitude of this disaster. The worst incidence of infant mortality in the United States in 1982 was in Washington, D.C., where 2 percent of all babies alive at birth died before their first birthdays. This high rate, almost double the U.S. average of 1.1 percent, was due in part to low birthweights and poor prenatal care in very young, often impoverished women. In Upper Volta, however, 21 percent of all infants die. More than 76 countries today endure infant mortality rates greater than 10 percent, and in regions of India and within some countries in Africa the rate exceeds 50 percent. These areas not only fare catastrophically worse than developed nations, but worse than several developing countries as well. China and Sri Lanka, despite income levels among the lowest in the world, have infant mortality rates of "only" 4 to 5 percent.[17] (See Table 2.) Low death rates have also been achieved in parts of India, Thailand, and Haiti, where primary health care procedures—midwifery, maternal education on breastfeeding and weaning, vaccinations, oral rehydration of victims of diarrhea, and antibiotics against respiratory infections—have been implemented.

Improved levels of female education also play a critical role in reducing infant mortality. Mothers with elementary training are taught how to avoid the causes of infant death, and they are better able to understand health workers' instructions. Primary health care can be fashioned to fit their needs and to help minimize the risks of catastrophic illness. Primary care, in a sense, can be considered an educational service.

Simply providing these most basic health care measures would save between five and ten million young lives each year. These services are most effective when delivered through a system of workers who can

Table 2: Infant Mortality and Female Literacy in Selected Countries

Country	Infant Mortality, 1981 (percent)	Female Literacy, 1980
Upper Volta	21	5
Afghanistan	20	6
Ethiopia	15	5
Bolivia	13	58
Nigeria	13	23
India	12	29
Pakistan	12	18
Saudi Arabia	11	12
Tanzania	10	23
Honduras	9	62
Brazil	8	73
Mexico	5	80
Philippines	5	88
Thailand	5	83
China	4.1	66
Yugoslavia	3.1	81
Costa Rica	2.7	92
Soviet Union	2.6	98
United States	1.2	99
Japan	0.7	99

Sources: United Nations Population Division; World Bank; and Ruth Leger Sivard, *World Military and Social Expenditures 1983* (Washington, D.C.: World Priorities, 1983).

give shots year after year at the required intervals, continuously teach breastfeeding and proper weaning, and provide birth control devices. Health workers with only limited training have cut infant mortality by half in demonstration projects, and for as little as $2 per person served per year. Extending primary health care to all of the world's peoples

> "In the Gambia,
> weight gain in pregnancy
> may average only six pounds."

would cost an additional $10 billion annually, one twenty-fifth as much as the world spends on cigarettes. Nevertheless, for many developing countries, this increase would require a doubling of health expenditures.[18]

Women and children in developing countries usually lack the most basic advantages. The Third World infant is disadvantaged even before birth because risk of death increases with low birth weight.[19] A Third World child's mother may gain only half as much weight in pregnancy as a woman in the developed world. During harvest seasons, when women must work exceptionally hard, or during rainy seasons, when food supplies are low, a childbearing woman may gain only a quarter as much weight as would be expected in the West. In the Gambia, weight gain in pregnancy during such difficult times may average only six pounds.[20] Women in food-short countries face not only scarcity along with everyone else, but usually receive low priority for food. A United Nations' survey showed that pregnant or lactating women throughout the Third World consume on average only 1750 calories per day, at least one-third fewer than recommended and one-third fewer than the men.[21] Often women in the developing world will be pregnant again after having lost a child only a few months earlier. Even when the last child has survived, a subsequent birth within 18 months and perhaps, as some research shows, even within 36 months, creates a significantly higher risk of infant mortality. The mother's system may not have fully recovered from the rigors of childbearing and she will be less able to gain weight and provide adequate milk.[22]

Half of all births in the Third World are delivered without any assistance from a trained midwife or doctor.[23] When midwives are available, a breech or otherwise complicated birth may be beyond their competence. In some areas, they may even cut the umbilical cord with a rusty razor and salve it with cow manure, a practice that contributes to the neonatal mortality caused by tetanus and infection in developing countries.[24]

If the child survives birth, it faces a treacherous year. The major threats include malnutrition due to poor weaning practices, diarrheal infection from contaminated water, and infectious diseases that prosper in malnourished children. Parents themselves frequently cause or permit malnutrition in their children. Children often become malnourished because infection depresses their appetites while it consumes additional calories. Common sense prompts parents to withhold food from a child infected with diarrhea because feeding increases stool volumes. The word diarrhea, in fact, means "to flow through." But the body still can use most of the food ingested during diarrhea, and so failure to feed children starves them unnecessarily. The resulting malnutrition then suppresses the body's immune responses. Repeated episodes of diarrhea, which are common where clean drinking water is unavailable, lead to further malnutrition, infection, and even death.

Dehydration caused by advanced diarrhea kills more dramatically. The large intestine normally absorbs salts and sugars through wall membranes using "pumps" in the cell membrane. Microorganisms such as Shigella dysentery produce toxins, shut down the pumps, or cause the membranes to excrete large quantities of fluids. Normally, the small intestine reabsorbs ten quarts of fluid per day, but diarrhea can reduce reabsorption to half this level. Dehydration follows, along with a high risk of death.[25]

Still another major disadvantage for children of the developing world is lack of access to medicine's most elegant solutions: vaccinations. Only one-third of these children are vaccinated against measles, for example. Inexpensive inoculations against the highly infectious and often deadly childhood diseases of whooping cough, diphtheria, and polio have been available for decades, but few Third World children receive them. Immunization campaigns have been attempted, but often yield poor results, in part because shots must be given to children over various intervals and to new infants year after year. Inadequate recordkeeping, refrigeration, and transportation each contribute to low participation in immunization campaigns.[26]

Different solutions for the health problems of the Third World are needed at each stage of life. Family planning services increase the chances of survival of all children. Parents in lands with high infant mortality rates typically produce more children than they desire because they have little access to contraception or because they want to

> "Family planning services increase the chances of survival of all children."

ensure the survival of a minimum number. Surveys have consistently shown that large numbers of Third World women desire birth control devices but do not have access to them.[27] Women fitted with IUD's or provided with birth control pills can space their children and limit their number.

Supplementing the food supply of pregnant women can provide cost-effective benefits. United Nations University (UNU) studies have shown that increasing calories, protein, iron, and other nutrients in the diets of pregnant women greatly enhances the survival of infants at birth by increasing birthweights. The UNU found these supplements far more beneficial than providing food to mothers for the purpose of increasing breastmilk production. Case studies of supplemental feeding of pregnant women, lactating mothers, infants, and children in Chile, India, Haiti, and Thailand also argue for giving pregnant women highest priority in any nutrition intervention efforts.[28] Health workers can monitor the weight of pregnant women and urge them—and urge their families to let them—eat more. Where heavy scales cannot be transported, simple tape measures for measuring arm circumference can help identify women with a high risk of giving birth to a low-weight child.[29]

Workers trained in midwifery can perform deliveries without infecting mother or child. Simply teaching traditional midwives to sterilize the razor blade used to sever the umbilical cord would help avoid neonatal infection. Similarly, inoculating pregnant women against tetanus would also provide immunity for the infant. Traditional midwives can be readily trained in delivery and vaccination methods. Training can be given on the job, thus avoiding a long and difficult absence from the village.

All primary care workers should be trained to promote breastfeeding; its advantages have been abundantly documented. Studies around the world have shown that artificially fed infants are several times more likely to contract diarrheal diseases and die. Healthy mothers can satisfy an infant's nutritional requirements through breastfeeding for at least six months and thus avoid the risk of infection carried by contaminated formulas or water. The colostrum, or foremilk, that flows from the mother's breasts immediately after birth is rich in antibodies that will protect the baby from diseases against which it otherwise would have little resistance. The milk itself is more nutritious than any substitute, and it is free—the money saved can be used to assure the nourishment of the mother. The importance of breastfeeding is obviously much more critical when clean water and sterile containers are unavailable for preparing formula.[30]

Failures in breastfeeding emphasize the need for promoting good weaning practices. Exclusive breastfeeding for many women is not practical for more than a few weeks. A survey in Barbados showed that 90 percent of all mothers believed breastfeeding to be superior, but only 45 percent breastfed fully at three months, and only 17 percent at six months. The gap between belief and behavior probably is due to the mother's need to work outside the home and a lack of daycare facilities near work. Neither problem can be readily or cheaply solved. In such circumstances, adequate weaning foods and clean water are essential.[31]

Weaning exposes infants to contaminated water and to unnourishing, indigestible foods. Unhealthy weaning practices throughout developing countries may explain why infant mortality is so high in nations where breastfeeding for long periods is common. Many Third World mothers may breastfeed even up to 18 months but supplement diets only with watery gruels or starches. Infants in the Third World are usually not fed adult foods, which are more nourishing, until they are five years old.[32] Health workers, as part of their routine visits to homes or in patients' visits to health centers, can teach families how to prepare foods that children can digest.

Simple tools are available to health workers to assure that infants and young children are being fed properly. Most malnourished children do not display the swollen stomach or wasted appearance that characterize severe malnutrition, and their parents may not know they are underfed. They may simply appear sickly or small for their age. By the time the condition is properly diagnosed, the child will be chronically ill and may soon die. Growth charts make obvious when additional food should be given. The charts, which cost 10 to 15 cents each, help a parent or a health worker compare the weight of children against "normal" weight for their age. If a child gains no weight for

> "Breast milk is more nutritious than any substitute."

three months, or falls below 65 percent of the norm, the chart will show that the child should receive additional food and perhaps other curative measures.[33]

Health workers are essential in treating diarrhea because they can show parents how and when to use oral rehydration therapy (ORT), a new technique that reduces dehydration due to diarrhea quickly and inexpensively. ORT has been successfully demonstrated among thousands of families in Guatemala, Honduras, Egypt, India, Bangladesh, and elsewhere, and has been credited with cutting infant mortality by half or more in these projects. Administering glucose in a given proportion with salts enhances intestinal absorption of fluids and halts their hyper-secretion. ORT packets can be manufactured for pennies per dose, or when packets are unavailable, workers can teach parents how to mix simple salt and sugar in correct proportions. Songs or inexpensive posters can help convey instructions to the illiterate. An essential part of the delivery of this service is instruction in early use, for delay can be fatal. Health workers can again make use of posters to display symptoms that call for administration of the tablets or mixture.[34]

The key to the delivery of these services is workers who are quickly trained, accepted by the community, willing to live in the area, and who serve without the great expense of highly trained doctors. The use of such workers—paramedics, "barefoot doctors," or whatever they may be called around the world—has been demonstrated by a few model primary health centers. Health worker systems in India, for example, have saved lives at a cost of about $60 to $75 per life saved.[35] The low cost reflects the use of workers with levels of education far below a physician's. Even though the cost of saving young lives may be several times higher in most of the Third World, primary health centers still are comparatively inexpensive.

A typical primary health care system works like the one in Dhende Mao, India, where a nurse with two years of government-sponsored training provides prenatal care, nutritional advice, vitamin supplements, inoculations, and antibiotics. The nurse is the middle level of a three-tier "health pyramid," and receives patients who cannot be helped by a first-aid nurse, usually a man who runs a fever treatment center in his home. If the first-aid nurse cannot help the people who come to him, he sends them to the nurse in the clinic. If she cannot help them either, she refers them to a doctor some 12 miles away.[36] This system of referrals facilitates treatment of the more difficult cases and enhances the system's credibility by also making the primary care workers providers of access to more sophisticated care.

A test of primary health care during the early seventies in Narangwal, India, has produced astonishing results. Three different experimental projects were conducted providing either medical care, nutrition supplements, or combined medical care and nutrition supplements. Similar villages nearby without significant primary health care services were studied for comparison and used as scientific "controls." The combined medical care and nutrition project reduced infant mortality to 7 percent compared to 13 percent in the control areas (70 per thousand versus 130 per thousand). The nutrition campaigns only reduced the infant death rate to 10 percent. The medical care only project, however, was cheapest and most effective in reducing child death and disease. Nutrition care cost $4.80 (1983 dollars) per person per year, compared to about $2.40 per person per year for medical care. Nutrition intervention targeted exclusively at pregnant women halved the stillbirth rate compared to the control group. The workers used in each of the Narangwal variations were mainly illiterate.[37] (See Table 3.)

Another project at Miraj, India, also conducted during the seventies, yielded similar results. With a per capita annual cost of only 85¢ per year, the results were impressive: Infant mortality was reduced in three years from 6.8 percent to 2.3 percent. The number of children immunized against the basic childhood diseases increased from about 5 percent to 85 percent for some vaccines. Ninety-seven percent of mothers received prenatal care. The birth rate was simultaneously reduced.[38]

Comparable results were obtained in a program in Haiti that used community health workers to expand the services available at the Albert Schweitzer Memorial Hospital. At the outset of the project, infant mortality was slightly lower in the countryside surrounding the hospital than the national average. But for less than $3.85 per person

Table 3: Primary Health Care Projects: Success Rates and Cost

Project	Infant Mortality Rate		Annual Cost Per Capita
	Project Area	Control Area	
	(percent)		(1983 dollars)
Guatemala, rural (1970-72)	5.5	8.5	$8.90
Haiti, rural (1968-72)	3.4	15.0	$3.85
India, Jamkhed (1971-76)	3.9	9.0	$1.55
India, Narangwal (1970-73)			
Medical care	7.0	12.8	$2.40
Nutrition Intervention	9.7	12.8	$4.80
Combined	8.1	12.8	$3.80
Nigeria, Imesi (1966-67)	4.8	9.1	$3.60

Sources: Davidson R. Gwatkin et al., *Can Health and Nutrition Interventions Make A Difference?* (Washington, D.C.: Overseas Development Council, 1980); Warren L. Berggren et al., "Reduction of Mortality in Rural Haiti Through A Primary-Health-Care Program," *The New England Journal of Medicine*, May 28, 1981; Rashid Faruqee and Ethna Johnson, "Health, Nutrition, and Family Planning in India," World Bank, February, 1982.

per year, rates of mortality were cut to one-sixth the national levels. Eighty-five percent of the children were inoculated for diphtheria, tetanus, and whooping cough, compared with only 15 percent nationally. Though literate, the workers employed did not have extensive education.[39]

These primary health care demonstration projects were also encouraging because local communities were involved in their operation and the projects became substantially self-supporting. Residents donated labor and materials. Charges assessed for curative services and medicines recovered up to 75 percent of operating costs. Those most in need of help, the very poor, were provided care free of charge, and were even sought out with home visits. These special efforts, as much as anything, led to the success of the projects. The combined practice of curative and preventive care—for male adults as well as women and children—thus made the system attractive and acceptable. Curative care filled a special need and made "community participation" meaningful.

18 A major achievement of primary health care projects has been a large increase in families practicing family planning. In Jamkhed, India, family planning participation rates increased from 10 percent in the surrounding area to 50 percent in the project. In the Miraj project, the rate increased from less than a third to almost 90 percent of the "eligible" couples. A couple's willingness to practice birth control strongly depended upon their past history of infant and child losses. As health care reduced the risk of having too few children survive, the number of parents using contraceptives increased quickly. Family planning was stimulated even in areas where sterilization campaigns had caused intense resentment.[40]

Findings from some prototype primary health care projects are discouraging. Government sponsored health-care projects in India, for example, did not achieve nearly the success rate as nongovernment projects, partly because the Indian government typically spent only one-fourth as much per primary health care center. A survey by the U.S. Agency for International Development of 52 primary care projects it funded showed that common problems include poor administration, lack of minimally educated personnel, lack of medicines and supplies, poor communication, poor transportation, and inadequate follow-up training—all formidable problems.[41]

Ghana and Thailand have experienced difficulties with their primary health care efforts. Lack of training in Ghana was blamed for the failure of nurse practitioners to even look inside childrens' throats for infection, to listen to their breathing, or to pinch the skin—a common test for dehydration in children with diarrhea. One doctor in Kenya bitterly denounced the concept of integrated primary services when adequate resources are not provided. "In theory integration provides everything," he wrote. "In reality it throws dust in the eyes of the public."[42] These experiences underscore the importance of individual initiative, good organization, flexibility, and planning in the success of primary health care. Primitive primary health care may only be an emergency measure taken in the tradition of triage. But it is the only

> "Average per capita expenditure on health for more than 2 billion people is only $1 to $2 per year."

practical prescription for hundreds of millions of children. To reduce infant mortality from 20 percent to 5 percent would represent a major improvement, even though this level would be considered intolerable in developed nations.

To achieve "health for all," the World Health Organization (WHO) has set as a goal the expenditure of 5 percent of each country's GNP on health care.[43] This may seem an odd target, for countries with low levels of income will require a far higher proportion of GNP to attain equivalent levels of health care as richer countries. But even the achievement of the WHO goal will require a major reorientation of development priorities. More than 76 countries—the most impoverished and the least healthy—spend less than 2 percent of their GNP on public health. Altogether, about 100 countries spend less than the WHO goal. This means that the average per capita expenditure on health for more than two billion people is only $1 to $2 per year, although private expenditures on traditional medicine may also equal this amount.[44] To meet the WHO goal by providing primary health care to 1.5 billion people without adequate services, an additional annual expenditure—or shift in expenditures—of about $7 per capita would be needed. This extra cost would total just over $10 billion per year. Moreover, half the budgets of the Ministries of Health in developing countries now go to hospitals that provide intensive care, mainly for upper-income urban dwellers. These nations will have to shift priorities within their current health care systems, unless they double or triple total health care spending.

Nations and multilateral aid institutions such as the World Bank have long spent more on energy, industrial, and transportation development than health. The World Bank's International Development Association, despite recent efforts in health investment, has invested over ten times as much money in energy as in health, nutrition, and family planning. The Agency for International Development, which funded primary health care and oral rehydration therapy in Thailand long before the 1978 international conference on primary health care in Alma-Ata, recently cut funding for its health activities by 20 percent. (This cut was prompted by the Reagan Administration's opposition to the family planning aspects of primary care.) The entire budget of the World Bank, in fact, is less than the $10 billion or so required to bring world health care up to even the most minimal levels.[45] Additional transfers—aid—from the rich countries are clearly needed. Meanwhile, developing nations themselves can elevate health on their investment agendas and use available resources more efficiently. Many Third World doctors cite the waste of resources in expensive hospitals that fail to provide the type of care that is most needed and perform large numbers of operations that may not be necessary.[46]

Health can become a central effort of nations only at the insistence of the needy citizens. Unfortunately, dissent is tolerated in only one-third of the world's nations. The importance of constructive criticism is plainly visible in all free lands, and the absence of civil liberties to promote such an exchange of ideas and the expression of political will is debilitating. The recent example of Somalia is indicative. Doctors and nurses there critical of the government's failure to accelerate the implementation of primary health care—they merely handed out leaflets to passers-by—were imprisoned without trial for four years.[47] Human health development requires the struggle for human rights. To the extent that powerful governments support oppressive regimes, there is a far greater cost in human life than just the lives lost in armed struggle.

Drinking Water and Toilets

Peter Bourne, president of Global Water, Inc., an organization formed to help implement the goals of the International Drinking Water Supply and Sanitation Decade, relates two stories that capture the meaning water carries for human health. The first comes from an African woman asked whether she understood the importance of encouraging her children to wash their hands after defecation, particularly before eating. She replied, "I have to carry our water seven miles every day. If I caught anyone wasting water by washing their hands, I would kill them." The second comes from another African woman asked how having water taps installed in her village had changed village life. Her immediate response was, "The babies no longer die."[48]

One-quarter of the world's people lack clean drinking water and sanitary human waste disposal. As a result, diarrheal diseases are endemic throughout the Third World and are the world's major cause of infant mortality. Cholera, typhoid fever, Guinea worm, schistosomiasis, and intestinal parasites also infect hundreds of mil-

Table 4: Principal Sources of Disease

Disease (common name)	Persons Infected (millions)	Controllable with Clean Water Supply and Basic Sanitation (percent)
Acquired In Drinking or Water Contact:		
Cholera	na	90
Typhoid Fever	na	80
Diarrhea	500[1]	50
Guinea Worms	na	100
Schistosomiasis	200	10
Acquired in Collecting Water:		
Malaria	300	na
Sleeping Sickness[2]	na	80
River Blindness	20-30	20
Elephantiasis[3]	270	na
Acquired by Contact with Excreta:		
Roundworm	650	40
Whipworms	350	na
Hookworms	450	na

[1] Estimate is for annual cases in children in developing countries. [2] Gambian Trypanosomiasis. [3] All Filariasis infection.

Sources: *Safe Water and Waste Disposal For Human Health: A Program Guide*, U.S. Agency for International Development, 1982; *Zoonoses And Communicable Diseases Common To Man and Animals* (Washington, D.C.: Pan American Health Organization, 1980).

lions. Many people, because they must visit rivers and swampy areas to obtain water, risk contracting malaria, river blindness, and sleeping sickness. Experts estimate that a sanitary water supply would eliminate half the diarrhea, including 90 percent of all cholera, 80 percent of sleeping sickness, and 100 percent of Guinea worm infestation, as well as smaller fractions of several other serious tropical diseases.[49] (See Table 4.)

Some observers have argued that water and sanitation systems should receive higher priority than other investments, including major reservoir projects, because they fundamentally improve the human condition, while some reservoirs have caused serous problems such as the tripling of cases of schistosomiasis. Clean drinking water, unfortunately, has not been a high priority for many countries. Four-fifths of the rural population of 73 African and Asian countries, where the populations are mostly rural, do not have access to clean drinking water. Most have no toilet or latrine. (See Table 5.) Worldwide, 1.3 billion people lack clean water and 1.7 billion lack adequate sanitation.[50]

Analysts at the World Bank have described the tragedy that follows failure in sanitation:

> A family lives in a palm-roofed, wooden house surrounded by rice fields and small irrigation channels, one of which, flowing near the house, serves as the domestic water supply. There are four children in the family; the mother has had six babies but one died following a sudden attack of diarrhea at the age of fifteen months, and a child of school age died in the cholera epidemic that swept through the area four years ago. . . . It is particularly difficult to control excreta in this damp environment; most feces are deposited not far from the house, and the younger children urinate in the canals nearby. Some years ago a government campaign was mounted to provide pit latrines, and one was dug near the family's house. They used it for a while, but in the monsoon season the pit flooded and a large quantity of fecal material was spread around the house. It was

Table 5: Availability of Clean Drinking Water and Human Waste Disposal in Selected Countries

Country	Infant Mortality	Share of Population with Service	
		Clean Drinking Water Supply	Human Waste Disposal
	(percent)	(percent)	
Upper Volta	21	31	na
Afghanistan	20	11	na
Angola	15	27	na
Ethiopia	15	16	14
Bolivia	13	37	24
India	12	42	20
Pakistan	12	34	6
Turkey	12	78	8
Indonesia	10	22	15
Tanzania	10	46	10
Honduras	9	44	20
Brazil	8	55	25
Mexico	5	57	28
Philippines	5	51	56
Chile	4.1	85	32
Costa Rica	2.7	72	97
Portugal	2.6	73	na
Soviet Union	2.6	76	na
Cuba	1.9	62	36
United States	1.2	99	99

Sources: *The State of the World's Children, 1984* (New York: Oxford University Press and the United Nations Children's Fund, 1983); Ruth Leger Sivard, "World Military and Social Expenditures, 1983," World Priorities, 1983; *Health Conditions in the Americas* (Washington, D.C.: Pan American Health Organization, 1982).

around that time that the cholera epidemic occurred, and its sad consequences for the family, together with the unpleasant mess, discouraged them from using the pit latrine again. . . . All the children get diarrhea several times a year, as do the parents from time to time. The worst occasion was when two daughters, both under three years of age, got it at the same time. The younger one seemed just to shrivel up overnight, and she died the next day.[51]

Last century in the United States and Great Britain, cholera and diarrhea rates dropped sharply, mainly because of improvements in sanitary conditions. Studies in California and Kentucky have shown that compared to disease rates for children with both indoor water and toilets, diarrhea occurred twice as often in children who had outside toilets and four times as often in children who had neither. In twenty American cities, the average reduction in typhoid fever following installation of water filtration was 65 percent. A Chilean study concluded that, "The availability of drinking-water . . . cut the incidence of acute diarrhea by about 74 percent." A case study in the Philippines found that toilet construction reduced cholera incidence by 70 percent. Privy construction in Costa Rica, according to the World Bank, helped cut the death rate in half for diarrhea and related diseases between 1942 and 1954.[52]

Both high cost and cultural barriers can easily block sanitation development. In Cameroon, for example, one toilet and drinking water project failed because capital costs exceeded the entire village's annual disposable income by 15 percent.[53] Even when construction is successfully completed, local attitudes may prevent the system from being used as designed. In Central America, one project failed because villagers felt the structures could be better used as chicken coops and grain bins. Similar obstacles have blocked progress in India. Villagers want water, but convenience is more important than quality. Food, housing, and fuel take precedence over water purity, and toilets are seen as a luxury, not a necessity.[54]

The engineering challenge comes in designing effective and inexpensive systems. Local materials must be used and social constraints

> "Privy construction in Costa Rica cut the death rate in half for diarrhea."

taken into consideration. Some toilet construction schemes have failed, for example, because the walls did not extend to the ground: women hesitated to use them because men could recognize their shoes. A problem of a different sort arose in Nairobi when the city required all housing to offer toilet facilities: the rule closed down low-income housing that owners deemed not worth the expense of improving.[55]

The design of water supply systems will vary according to local conditions. Surface water supply, cisterns, hand-dug, hand-driven, or deep, hydraulically drilled wells may be required. Though well developed, the various technologies can be prohibitively expensive when delivered on a large scale. Large drill rigs are not only expensive to buy and operate, but difficult to transport over poor roads. More adaptable are small, jeep-mounted rigs capable of drilling to a depth of 100 feet. Hand-dug wells can be sunk into soft soils with high water tables at a very low cost. Labor can be provided by those who will use the well, and the only materials required are concrete, reinforcing bars, and wood for a cover and pump or windlass. Simple wells will work as long as groundwater is not contaminated by human or animal feces, and if the wellhead is designed to prevent contamination. For example, a child with Guinea worm can easily infect the well if he or she steps in the water, for the female worms lay eggs under the skin where they form blisters that burst when immersed. Even bucket wells are subject to contamination by careless handling. Placing the bucket on the ground, or handling it with dirty hands, will contaminate the water and infect the well's other users. This problem may account for the failure of wells to reduce diarrhea in some communities.[56]

Driven wells, pipes hammered into the ground by a person using a sledgehammer, can be sunk up to 45 feet. The system requires a pump and must be inexpensive, reliable, and easy to repair locally. Spring or gravity-fed systems work well, but only when the water supply is elevated above potential human or animal contamination. Springs in particular require covers to prevent contamination at the point of collection. In Malawi, a highly successful gravity-fed system distributes water over a 90-mile distance—without a single moving part.[57]

Table 6: Cost of Minimal Levels of Water Supply

Water Supply	Total Investment Cost Per Capita	
	Urban	Rural
	(1983 dollars)	
House connection	120	150
Standpipe	40	40
Hand pumps	—	25

Source: "Water Supply and Waste Disposal," World Bank, 1983.

Much of the poor hygiene in the Third World is due to the sheer difficulty of moving water, which weighs about eight pounds per gallon, not counting the container. For adequate hygiene, people need about four or five gallons per day. For each individual, this means carrying 40 pounds of water each day. If the burden for supplying water to a family of seven falls to the mother and daughters, as usually happens, they share the back-breaking job of carrying over 300 pounds of water per day. Then follows the hard work of bathing children, cooking, and cleaning. Thus, they fall behind in the fight against the pathogens in their environments.

Easing this burden will require sizable capital investments. The World Bank estimates that village water supply systems, assuming the installation of public standpipes to be shared among approximately 140 persons, would cost $20 to 40 per capita depending on the size of the village. (See Table 6.) Surface water, even if turbid or contaminated, can be treated, made potable, and delivered through public standpipes for as little as $40 per capita. The costs include sand filters to remove amoeba cysts that cause dysentery and chlorination to kill any bacterial contamination.[58]

The World Bank estimates that indoor water and sanitation for the Third World would cost $800 billion to construct and $10 billion per year to operate and maintain.[59] Thus, as with water supply, only inexpensive excrement disposal systems will be practical in the devel-

Table 7: Cost of Minimal Levels of Human Waste Disposal

Low-Cost Toilets	Cost Per Household		Share of Income of Average Low-income Household
	Total Investment	Hypothetical Total Per Month	
	(1983 dollars)		(percent)
Pour-flush toilet	$ 70	$2.0	2
Pit latrine	$125	$2.6	3
Communal toilet	$355	$8.3	9
Vacuum-truck cartage	$105	$3.8	4
Vietnamese Toilet	$ 50	—	—

Sources: "Water Supply and Waste Disposal," World Bank, 1983; *Human Waste Management For Low-Income Settlements* (Bangkok: Environmental Sanitation Information Center, 1983).

oping countries. Fortunately, several appropriate technologies are available and affordable. (See Table 7.)

One inexpensive substitute for indoor toilets, the Vietnamese toilet, combines functional sophistication and technical simplicity. It consists of an intake that separates urine and feces and two above-ground concrete chambers, used alternately, that anaerobically digest human waste. Because the system is sealed, it can be used in flood-prone or high water table areas. Pouring ashes into the chambers promotes decomposition and makes the waste suitable as a fertilizer within a year. The separated urine travels to an ash-filled container and remains for a few days, after which it can be used as fertilizer. This system is reportedly used widely in Vietnam, and it has also been introduced in Tanzania, Mozambique, and elsewhere.[60]

The more widely used aqua-privy is a single tank, partly filled with water, into which human waste is carried via a drop-pipe. The system is "sealed" by a layer of scum on the water surface that keeps odors in, allowing breakdown of waste without oxygen. The drop-pipe extends below the water line from either a squatting plate or a pedestal that can be flushed with two or three liters of water. An overflow outlet, also submerged, carries effluent underground, and so the toilet must be well above the water table. Digested materials can be removed periodically by the owner.[61]

The aqua-privy has been widely installed in India, largely through citizens' efforts and local entrepreneurs such as Bindeshwar Pathak. These citizens deplored the conditions in which "scavengers," the Bhangi caste, had to remove fresh night soil daily, often carrying the material on their heads in poorly constructed containers. Efforts to halt this practice, along with the backing of Prime Minister Indira Gandhi, led to legislation in several Indian states requiring the installation of aqua-privies. Both state grants and loans were made to install the privies, and special financing permitted buyers to pay off their loans over a two-year period without interest. Buyers also received a five-year guarantee and a free first cleaning.[62]

Less sophisticated systems, including the cesspool used widely in Thailand and the simple pit privy used around the globe, can create serious problems.[63] Though acceptable in some areas, they carry considerable risk of failure from flooding. Expertise is needed to install the systems, either from government agencies, health workers, or private entrepreneurs. Projects seem to work best when citizens are taught to construct and operate their own systems. Primary health care workers can make sure the facilities are used properly, but governments are usually organized so that sanitation projects are administered by an agency other than the Ministry of Health. Separate responsibility for health care need not be counterproductive, as long as the two efforts are coordinated.

Coordination between sanitary engineering and health maintenance makes sense because sanitation will both reduce the cost of health care and promote economic efficiency. Health care services could serve as an incentive to install and use sanitation facilities; curative services could be discounted for those who comply. To assure compliance, health or sanitation workers would have to visit households to check the operation and maintenance of the toilets and latrines. Health

> "Sanitation projects work best when citizens are taught to construct and operate their own systems."

workers could do this during home visits to deliver preventive and curative care.

Demonstration programs offer a cost-effective way to promote sanitary methods. One model program of large-scale public education through hands-on demonstrations was created by the Tennessee Valley Authority (TVA). Though TVA promoted agriculture and not sanitation, the model itself is instructive. TVA selected locally respected farmers willing to try a new idea—fertilizer use—and provided free fertilizer to those who agreed to use it for five years and publicize their experiences in local seminars.[64] Water and sanitary methods can be demonstrated the same way, involving a single family, a neighborhood, or an entire village. World Bank analyst Colin Glennie, describing the value of demonstrations as an educational tool, said, "Target communities who are able to see the results of an initial project, and who can talk to the beneficiaries, will be far more impressed than they could ever be by listening to Government propaganda or the exhortations of their leaders."[65]

The importance of support from government leaders cannot be underestimated. In India, backing from Indira Ghandi for aqua-privies was merely symbolic, but with her endorsement, many of the barriers, both psychological and bureaucratic, came down. Because sanitary efforts will be expensive, leaders will be called on to make available greater resources than now are being applied. The investments will, at an acceptable cost, vastly improve human health and resources.[66]

Low-risk Diets

Heart disease and cancer cause two-thirds of all deaths in the developed world, a third of which occur before age sixty-five. Though formerly associated with affluence, these diseases have grown more serious throughout the world. The combined cost of medical care and lost economic productivity due to heart disease and cancer approaches $100 billion per year in the United States alone. Coronary by-pass surgery can increase the chance of survival of heart disease by 50 percent, but at a cost of $20,000 per procedure. Chemotherapy and surgery for some types of cancer also can lengthen life, but cost large sums of money. Recent evidence that heart disease and cancer are associated with diet, particularly fats and cholesterol, has raised hope that early death due to these diseases can be substantially prevented, and that their economic costs can be greatly reduced.[67] Some experts, however, remain skeptical that preventive medicine can reduce the toll of heart disease and cancer because changing people's habits is difficult, screening for high-risk individuals can be expensive, and dietary prescriptions are complex.

The bewildering complexity of cancer and heart disease has led many to despair of avoiding these catastrophic diseases. Heart disease has been linked to the very foods people in the developed world have been taught are most wholesome: eggs, beef, and dairy products. Reports seem to come daily that everything from mushrooms to peanut butter causes cancer. Indeed, human metabolism itself may with age lead inevitably to these diseases. But cancer and heart disease rates vary widely around the world, a fact that suggests they can be reduced. The risk of breast cancer, for example, is more than four times greater for an American woman than for a Japanese woman, possibly because the American diet contains two to four times as many calories from fat as the Japanese diet. Japanese who move to the United States and adopt American eating habits develop rates of colon and breast cancer similar to the Americans. Fat consumption and cancer of the colon and breast, the two leading cancer killers after lung cancer, show high statistical correlation internationally. This correlation holds despite differences among countries in other suspected causes of cancer, including uses of industrial chemicals, energy, and non-diet lifestyles. Diets high in fiber and vitamins E and A (or its precursor, β-Carotene) seem to protect against colon cancer. Diets high in pickled and salt-preserved foods, including those of Scandinavians and Japanese, seem to increase stomach cancer. Diets of poorly preserved foods, common in Africa, increase the risk of liver cancer because the powerful carcinogen aflatoxin is produced in these foods by bacteria. Westerners are exposed to aflatoxin in peanut butter, but their low rates of liver cancer suggest that their overall risk due to this factor is low. Studying variations such as these, epidemiologists Richard Doll and Richard Peto, in a landmark study published in 1981, estimated that 35 to 50 percent of all cancers, in the

> "The risk of breast cancer is more than four times greater for an American woman than a Japanese woman."

United States, at least, could some day be avoided by adherence to dietary guidelines.[68] (See Table 8.)

The risk of heart disease also correlates with dietary habits. Heart attack rates among U.S. immigrants from Japan, where consumption of saturated fat and cholesterol is low, climb as they adopt U.S. diets. This trend, which correlates with low heart attack rates among U.S. vegetarians, suggests that people with high cholesterol levels could reduce their risk of heart attack by reducing their cholesterol levels. A recently completed ten-year test of this theory in the United States showed that a 1 percent reduction in blood cholesterol levels produced a 2 percent reduction in heart attack risk. These results suggest that overall heart attack rates in the United States could be reduced up to 50 percent by a 25 percent reduction in cholesterol blood levels.[69]

Better understanding of the biochemistry of heart disease and cancer has given credence to the theories that diet substantially contributes to their development. Cholesterol, an essential component of cell walls and the raw material for hormone production in the body, is manufactured in the human liver and ingested in meat, dairy products, and eggs. The liver's daily production of cholesterol of between 500 and 1000 milligrams per day is somewhat reduced by dietary cholesterol consumption, but is increased in response to saturated fats consumption.[70]

Coronary heart disease is primarily the result of cholesterol plaque buildup in the arteries that supply blood to heart muscle. The disease is defined by the obstruction of at least 50 percent of this blood supply, and heart attack results when insufficient oxygen reaches the heart muscle, causing injury or death of the muscle cells. Age, male sex, hypertension, cigarette smoking, and diabetes are major risk factors for coronary heart disease along with diet.[71] Blocked arteries can also lead to a cerebral stroke (though stroke is more frequently caused by hemorrhage). Cholesterol plaques block the flow of blood and oxygen to the brain, usually by obstructing the carotid artery where it branches in the neck. Surgeons have removed cholesterol plaques from the carotid as thick as an inch and as long as two inches.[72]

Table 8: Sources of Risk for Contracting Cancer, United States

Cause or Risk Factor	Sites Affected	Portion of Cancers (percent)
Diet	Colon, Breast, Uterus, Ovary	35 - 50
Tobacco	Lung, Esophagus, Bladder, Kidney, Pancreas	22 - 30
Occupation, asbestos	Lung, others	3 - 18
Occupation, all exposures	Lung, other	4 - 38
Alcohol	Stomach, Larynx, Liver	3 - 5
Infection	Cervix, Prostate, others	1 - 15
Sexual development and practices	Breast, Uterus, Ovary, Cervix, Testis	1 - 13
Pollution	Lung, Bladder, Rectum	3 - 5
Medicines and radiation	Breast, Uterus, Ovary, Thyroid, Bone, Lung, Blood	1 - 4
Natural radiation	Skin, Breast, Thyroid, Lung, Bone, Blood	1 - 3
Consumer products	Possibly all sites	1 - 2

Note: Percentages will not add to 100 because of the uncertainty implicit in each estimate, and because some cancers have multiple causes.

Source: Adapted from U.S. Congress Office of Technology Assessment, *Assessment of Technologies for Determining Cancer Risks From the Environment* (Washington, D.C.: U.S. Government Printing Office, 1981).

Cancer is a multiple-stage process involving mutagens, or initiators, and promoters. An initiator alters the genetic code in a cell and creates the potential for cancer development. A promoter may help cause cancer in one or more ways: increasing the likelihood of cancer formation by interfering with a cell's process for repairing errors in DNA replication; accelerating the reproduction of tissue, thus prompting cell replication before repair can be completed; or facilitating the movement of mutagens into proximity with cell DNA. Tobacco and

> "Almost no correlation exists between the amount of fat and cholesterol in many common foods."

rancid or metabolized fat may serve as both initiators and promoters of cancer. Alcohol, though not an initiator, is a strong promoter of cancer of the esophagus initiated by tobacco use.[73]

Some scientists argue that industrial chemicals and pollutants have increased cancer rates, though others maintain that overall cancer rates have been constant for the last century. Industrial carcinogens and some food additives continue to be major public health problems, however. Such substances may be associated with only 5 percent of U.S. cancers, but this fraction represents 40,000 new cases of cancer each year.[74] Banning the use of these chemicals may cause little economic burden to society as a whole, for noncarcinogenic substitutes usually can be found. But the confirmation of carcinogens can be costly, as the definitive test for carcinogenicity costs at least $600,000 per chemical, and over 60,000 chemicals are currently in commercial use. Only a few hundred of these have been tested.[75] The control of chemical and occupational carcinogens will remain a high priority even as attention is turned to dietary factors as major risks.

The connection between fat consumption and cancer remains statistical: a causal relationship has not been proven. The association is so strong, however, and the benefits of minimizing fat consumption so beneficial for heart disease, weight control, diabetes prevention, and self-image, that reducing fat consumption can safely, even urgently, be recommended.[76] Unfortunately, few people can determine how much fat, cholesterol, or for that matter, how much salt, calories, and other foods with health risks they consume. The prescription for preventing both heart disease and cancer is in some ways similar. Eating meat increases both fat and cholesterol intake, and so substituting other sources of protein can reduce risk for both diseases. Almost no correlation exists, however, between the amount of fat and cholesterol in many common foods prepared from animal products. Some are high in one and low in the other. Foods prepared from vegetable products contain no cholesterol, but some contain both saturated and unsaturated fat.[77]

Promoting low-risk diets poses many difficulties. The risk associated with fat consumption, for example, is a function of the percent of total calories provided by fat, and calorie requirements vary by sex, age, and activity. Nutritionists caution against blanket statements such as "Don't eat eggs," even though eggs account for 45 percent of the cholesterol ingested by Americans.[78] For some vegetarians, the old, and the poor, eggs are properly a major source of essential protein. Cholesterol consumption is far less of a problem in people with low-fat diets.

A more serious problem is that cholesterol and fat are often hidden in foods. Many products such as breads, cakes, pies, casseroles, and other dishes contain eggs and butter. Even a single egg per day, hidden or not, provides the maximum recommended allowance of cholesterol for most Westerners. Furthermore, restricting certain foods can lead to nutritionally unbalanced diets. To some extent, screening for high-risk individuals and providing them with dietary advice can ease these problems.

Screening for high-risk individuals—people with elevated blood pressure or serum cholesterol levels—would help identify people most in need of dietary changes, and would also provide the motivation—reduced risk of catastrophic illness—to change. High blood pressure, for example, is the single best indicator of risk for heart disease, and screening for victims permits preventive treatment. The risk that a 35-year-old man will have a heart attack before age 55 doubles when his blood pressure increases from 120/80 to 142/90. The risk of having a stroke for a 45-year-old man increases tenfold when the lower figure in a blood pressure reading is above 104. A U.S. government campaign to increase awareness of the danger of hypertension has helped identify 8 to 10 million people with high blood pressure and provide them with treatment, including medicines that control hypertension and diets low in salt and other risks. Now over 80 percent of all Americans over 45 years of age have annual blood pressure tests, an increase of 25 percent since 1974. The success of this campaign suggests that a similar one could succeed for screening of cholesterol levels.[79]

Screening as a preventive measure can be quite expensive, however. One study suggested that each year of life extended in the United States by the blood pressure effort costs over $20,000. Several reasons account for this high cost, including the requirement that screening

> "Cholesterol consumption has dropped by 10 percent in the United States."

measures be provided to a much larger population than will actually benefit. Also, screening must be performed years in advance of the benefit, thus diverting health resources from other measures that might save an equal number of lives but over a shorter time. Finally, there is no guarantee that all or even most of the high-risk persons identified will follow the dietary prescriptions.[80]

But evidence is growing that preventive nutrition, coupled with screening for high-risk individuals, can be effective. The U.S. death rate has dropped 33 percent for heart disease and 44 percent for stroke since 1970. Both preventive and curative measures contributed to this success. Better emergency treatment helped reduce the rate of those dying of heart attacks before reaching a hospital by 25 to 30 percent. The blood pressure screening campaign no doubt contributed. But saturated fat and cholesterol consumption also dropped by 5 percent and 10 percent, respectively, between 1967 and 1982. Some of this change must be credited to public information campaigns conducted through the media by the government and public health organizations such as the American Heart Association. Similar efforts in Belgium have reduced heart disease there, though no comparable successes have been reported elsewhere in Europe. Tempering the U.S. success, however, is the fact that as saturated fat consumption declined, unsaturated fat consumption increased to the extent that total fat consumption—and the risk of cancer—increased slightly.[81]

The dietary education campaigns in the United States to date have been quite modest. The U.S. National Cancer Insitute, for example, recently launched a campaign to educate Americans about the risk of tobacco and fat consumption. But its advertising and publications budget for this campaign amounts to just one-tenth of one percent of the tobacco industry's annual advertising budget.[82]

Public education programs can be designed to fit most nutritional problems, and recommended daily allowances can provide an inexpensive and valuable guide to safe nutrition. Preventive medicine can be made a part of basic education, and thus moved out of the more expensive medical realm. Schools can teach children in detail about their dietary requirements, the composition of foods, and the risks associated with high consumption of fats and cholesterol. Nutrition education will have to be tailored to each country's situation, of course. In Japan, for example, where fat accounts for only 10 to 15 percent of calories, recommended levels of fat consumption can be lower than those made in the United States. In both the United States and Norway, fat accounts for more than 40 percent of calories. Limiting fat intake to 30 percent of daily caloric consumption in these countries may be a more practical recommendation. Where people traditionally rely on vegetable protein, recommendations can be set lower.

General outlines of good dietary practice, and even detailed instruction in schools, will still leave many without knowing what to do. More specific information is needed—as an aid to those instructed in safe nutrition as well as those beyond school age. Easy-to-interpret labels for food products would provide the foundation for safer diets. Some foods are already labled for fat, cholesterol, and calories, as well as vitamins, but this is voluntary and is usually provided in terms of total grams or ounces. To be useful, people have to translate these terms into minimum and maximum allowances, although recommended daily allowances (RDAs) are sometimes provided for vitamins. Recommended daily allowances (maximum) for fat and cholesterol would greatly help people plan their meals. The National Cancer Institute provides information to help estimate fat and cholesterol levels, but printing estimates right on food containers would be far more effective.

Under a more comprehensive labeling system, a package of very lean hamburger might carry the label, "Each four ounce serving contains 6 percent for males and 8 percent for females of the recommended daily maximum allowance of fat, and 33 percent for males and 44 percent for females of the recommended daily maximum allowance for cholesterol." An egg carton would state that one serving—one egg—provides 84 and 112 percent for males and females, respectively, of the recommended daily maximum allowance for cholesterol. The consumer could then easily see that eating an egg for breakfast and a hamburger for lunch exceeds the daily recommended cholesterol limit, and that a continuous diet of that type carries serious risk for heart disease.[83] (See Table 9.)

Table 9: Illustration of Labeling Foods For Health Risks, Maximum Daily Allowance, Selected Items

Item	Cholesterol		Fat[2]	
	Male	Female	Male	Female
	(percent)			
Beef Liver (3 oz.)	124	165	10	13
Egg (1)	84	112	6	8
Shrimp (3 oz.)	43	57	1	1
Steak (4 oz.)	70	92	40	55
Beef Hot Dog (3 oz.)	25	33	18	24
Chicken (white meat, 3 oz.)	24	32	5	6
Hamburger (3 oz.)	33	44	6	8
Butter (1 tbsp.)	10	14	12	17
Margarine (1 tbsp.)	0	0	12	17
Whole Milk (1 cup)	11	15	9	12
Skim Milk (1 cup)	1	2	1	1
Ice Cream (1 cup)	18	24	15	21
Spaghetti, meat sauce, and garlic bread[1]	83	113	52	66
2 eggs, 2 bacon slices, 2 pieces of toast[1]	185	246	35	47
Quiche Lorraine	61	81	35	47
Potato with margarine	0	0	6	7

[1] Packages containing ingredients of common dishes could be labeled for the RDA of the dish; recipes can also describe RDAs. [2] Recommended maximum for the United States in the immediate future. Long-term recommendation, and recommendation in countries where fat consumption can more easily be reduced or kept low, can be a third lower.

Source: Worldwatch Institute. See Note 83.

Some food manufacturers will have a strong interest in making such information available about their product and will—many already do—provide it willingly. Many others, however, will find their sales reduced by the provision of the data, and so will not provide it unless it is made a uniform requirement.[84] As if to illustrate the failure of institutions to evolve to meet human needs, the U.S. Department of Agriculture, despite recent revisions, still grades and labels meats on the basis of fat content, because high fat connotes flavor. The higher the fat, the higher the grade.

Some analysts remain pessimistic that screening and proscriptive dietary measures will be as cost-effective as emergency hospital coronary care units or basic research, for example. They recommend a lower priority for preventive measures. Studies of the cost-effectiveness of prevention, however, typically equate the quality of life after a heart attack with quality of life in a person who avoided a heart attack. Since activity is severely reduced for a year or longer after a heart attack, this is obviously fallacious.[85] As Louise Russell, an economist at the Brookings Institution points out, these economic analyses take a narrow perspective by assuming that screening can be performed only in medical facilities and early in life. The analyses, moreover, typically discount future benefits at a rate higher than private sector profits, also an assumption hard to defend.[86]

Preventive measures may not, in fact, cut total medical costs as advocates often claim, for when people live longer they may require more medical care than otherwise, thus increasing total costs.[87] Avoiding the cost of lost wages and economic productivity, however, does justify major expenditures on prevention. For example, a preventive measure costing $50 per person would pay for itself twelve times over if it avoided just 1 percent of all fatal heart attacks before age sixty-five.[88] Screenings for blood pressure and even cholesterol, moreover, are now routinely performed outside the medical sector, and cost very little. Nutrition education conducted in schools should add very little to total educational costs.

Preventive measures, though perhaps not a panacea for health care costs, can be readily justified in a broader context of economic efficiency and human welfare. For those willing to act on information, preventive nutrition offers longer, more productive lives.

Anti-smoking Measures

Many medical experts consider cigarette smoking the largest single preventable health problem in the developed world, and warn that it is becoming epidemic in the developing world. Cigarette smoking is believed responsible for one-third of all cancers, including three-fourths of all lung cancer in men. Most emphysema, bronchitis, half of all asthma and ulcers, and one-fifth of all heart attacks have been attributed to smoking. The overall health cost of smoking in the United States, including productivity losses as well as direct health expenditures, exceeds $40 billion each year, or $2 per pack of cigarettes. (See Table 10.) People in the United States spend $22 billion annually to buy cigarettes and worldwide spending totals an estimated $250 billion.[89]

Table 10: Estimated Human and Economic Costs of Smoking, United States, 1980

Disease	Lives Lost	Economic Cost
		(billion dollars)
Cancer	93,000	11
Cardiovascular	158,000	15
Digestive	12,000	8
Respiratory	25,700	8
Total	289,000	42

Source: Dorothy P. Rice and Thomas A. Hodgson, "Economic Costs of Smoking: An Analysis of Data For The United States," draft report presented at the Allied Social Science Association Annual Meetings, San Francisco, December 28, 1983.

Smoking will kill one in four of all smokers, mainly through heart disease and cancer. Smoking precipitates heart attacks by decreasing the oxygen content of the blood. Carbon monoxide absorbed from cigarette smoke displaces oxygen in the blood, thus increasing the volume needed to deliver a given amount of oxygen. Combined with atherosclerosis, which restricts blood flow in the coronary arteries, smoking can easily lead to a catastrophic oxygen shortage in the heart muscle, what is called a heart attack. Smokers who increase their carbon monoxide level to 5 percent increase the risk of heart attack by twentyfold. The carbon monoxide level of passive smokers—those who do not themselves smoke but who involuntarily inhale smoke from others—has been measured at 2 to 3 percent. The carbon monoxide content in the blood of heavy smokers reaches 15 percent.[90]

In cancer, smoking serves as both an initiator—that is, causes a mutation in a cell's genetic code that can lead to cancer—and a promoter. Cigarettes contain several substances that are mutagenic, including radioactivity and tar, that attack the membrane of the bronchus and the lung. Tumors may also develop when the tissues lining the bronchus and lung are damaged. Cigarettes are thus a complete carcinogen. Pipe and chewing tobacco also are carcinogenic.[91]

Worldwide tobacco consumption has increased considerably over the last ten years and continues to climb at a rate of 1 percent each year. Cigarette smoking is growing most rapidly in developing countries, increasing during the seventies by 4 to 6 percent annually in Brazil, India, and Pakistan, and 8 percent each year in Kenya. Fifty-five to 80 percent of adult males smoke in areas of Nepal, Senegal, Bangladesh, and China. Smoking among adult males in the United Kingdom has declined from 75 percent in 1962 to 50 percent, and in the United States the total is only 38 percent and falling.[92]

Efforts to control tobacco consumption have included education, health warnings, prohibition of advertising, and restriction of smoking in public places. A few countries have taken each step, while most have only the mildest restrictions, or none of them. (See Table 11.)

Anti-smoking efforts led by the Royal College of Physicians since 1962 in the United Kingdom and by the U.S. Surgeon General since 1964

Table 11: Cigarette Consumption, Taxes, and Control Policies, Selected Countries

Country	Tax per Pack (percent)	Warning	Advertising Restrictions	Annual Cigarette Consumption Per Capita[1] (number)
Argentina	70	None	None	1190
Brazil	70	None	Mild	1040
Chile	73	Mild	None	770
China	150-250	None	None	900
Costa Rica	8	Mild	None	870
Egypt	na	Strong	Prohibited	870
France	71	Mild	Mild	1610
India	70	Mild	None	120
Japan	55	None	Moderate	2600
Mexico	58	None	None	na
Nigeria	15-45	None	None	130[2]
Senegal	37[3]	Strong	Prohibited	na
United Kingdom	75	Mild	Mild	1820
United States	23	Mild	Moderate	2680
West Germany	46	Mild	Mild	1870
Zimbabwe	55	na	Strong	440

[1] This figure is the average for everyone, men, women, and children. [2] Cigarette consumption is particularly sensitive to income in poor countries. [3] Estimate.

Sources: Compiled by the Worldwatch Institute from "Tariff and Non-Tariff Measures on Tobacco," U.S. Department of Agriculture, 1984; and Royal College of Physicians, *Health or Smoking?* (London: Pitman Publishing Ltd., 1983).

helped halt the growth in cigarette use in those countries and reverse it. The U.S. campaign is credited with saving an estimated 200,000 lives between 1964 and 1984. Twenty times this number, however, almost 4 million people, died of smoking-related diseases over the same period in the United States alone.[93]

42 Many people, even in the United States and United Kingdom, still claim to be unaware of the hazards of smoking and the benefits of quitting. A survey in 1979 found that about half of U.S. smokers said they did not know that smoking causes most cases of lung cancer. Thirty-one percent claimed not to know that smoking contributes significantly to the risk of heart attack. In a recent survey, 30 percent of all British smokers denied that smoking harms their health. A much smaller number knew that smoking is dangerous, even if kept below 20 cigarettes per day, or that quitting would appreciably reduce health risks. Despite a mild warning on cigarette packs and occasional reports of new evidence that smoking is harmful, the United Kingdom is still far short of its official goal of eliminating smoking.[94] The U.S. Congress has recently moved to strengthen the health warning on cigarette packs and in advertising.

A major reason for public confusion over smoking is tobacco advertising. Tobacco companies spend about three-quarters of a billion dollars per year in U.S. magazines and newspapers, more than is spent to advertise any other product, including automobiles.[95] Cigarette manufacturers target vulnerable groups, regularly dispensing free samples of cigarettes, for example, to college students on spring vacation at crowded beaches. Their advertising emphasizes youth, virility, and sophistication. People in developing countries are told that smoking is "the modern thing to do." Phrases such as "Alive With Pleasure" on cigarette billboards are obvious double-entendres.[96]

Only a few countries prohibit cigarette advertising, including Finland, Norway, Egypt, and Senegal. In the United States, cigarette advertising is allowed in newspapers, magazines, and on billboards, but not on radio or television. The ban followed a government policy in the early seventies requiring radio and television to provide free air time to anti-smoking groups equal to one-fourth of paid tobacco advertising. Cigarette manufacturers consented to a ban on all advertising over the airwaves in order to avoid the anti-smoking messages.

> "The learning ability of eleven-year-olds whose mothers smoke has been reduced by six months."

The price of tobacco and its relation to income largely explains the variation in tobacco use around the world. Recent cigarette price increases, mostly due to government taxes, have a direct effect on consumption. Excise taxes on tobacco in the United Kingdom amount to more than 75 percent of the retail price, much higher than the U.S. rate of about 27 percent. As a result, even though more Britains smoke, consumption averages 30 to 40 percent lower than in the United States. Anti-smoking activists in the United States have urged that cigarettes be taxed at $2 per pack, equal to the health and productivity losses to society as a whole. Such a tax, they argue, not only would place the burden for the cost of smoking on smokers, but would provide them a strong incentive to quit. More important, a heavy tax would discourage young people from picking up the habit.[97] In developing countries, where treatment for smoking-related diseases requires already limited health care resources, taxing tobacco could be particularly effective.

Few countries require more than mild health warnings on cigarette packs. Mexico, though it imposes a tax of about 80 percent of the retail price of cigarettes, requires only an innocuous warning. South Korea outlaws foreign-made cigarettes, but more to reduce expensive imports and foreign debt than improve health, as locally produced cigarettes are promoted. Several countries still require no warnings or restrictions on tobacco use. Ethiopia, Mali, Malawi, Nigeria, Guyana, Argentina, Brazil, Paraguay, Indonesia, and Nepal require no warnings whatsoever. Of this group, Brazil and Argentina impose heavy taxes on tobacco, but the rest do not.[98]

The adverse health effects of smoking on nonsmokers have now been clearly established, especially for pregnant women. Lung cancer appears to be higher among nonsmoking wives of heavy smokers in Japan. The learning ability of eleven-year-olds whose mothers smoke has been shown to be reduced by six months. And workers who involuntarily breathe cigarette smoke are exposed to the equivalent of up to 6 cigarettes per day.[99]

In the last few years, some state and local governments have moved to protect the health and comfort of nonsmokers from the smoke of others. In the United States, Arizona, Minnesota, San Francisco, and

Alexandria, Virginia, restrict smoking in most enclosed public places and require employers to accommodate any worker who requests a smoke-free workplace. In Minnesota, a third of all restaurant seats must be set aside for nonsmokers. Several businesses in the United States have voluntarily forbidden smoking on the job by their employees. Their motivation is safety, savings on health insurance and disability costs, and reduced sick leave and employee inefficiency.[100]

Health education in schools and campaigns in the media to discourage smoking have proved effective. Prohibition of all tobacco advertising has been shown to be a particularly effective anti-smoking measure in Norway, where a ban enacted in 1971 sharply cut cigarette consumption. Also important are unambiguous warnings on tobacco products that smoking, even moderately, vastly increases the risk of heart disease and cancer.

Smoking can be discouraged by taxation, particularly among the young and in developing countries. A tax of $2 per pack in the United States can be justified because smoking costs society that amount in health care expenses and productivity losses. In developing countries, where health care resources are already severely strained, an even higher tax could be justified, as could other measures such as restrictions on imports. Because cigarettes are usually imported, and use is highest among the rich, cigarette use in developing lands presents a serious equity issue. Smoking requires more health resources for the rich and places additional burdens on scarce foreign exchange.

All countries can protect workers from cigarette smoke in the workplace. Laws restricting public smoking will strongly reinforce the growing belief, in developed countries at least, that smoking is socially unacceptable, a crucial attitude in reducing smoking.

Finally, smokers should receive help in withdrawing from cigarette dependence. Over two-thirds of all U.S. smokers have tried to quit and failed. "How-to-quit" sessions can be profitable, especially for employers who would gain increased productivity and reduced disability and health insurance costs. Preliminary evidence indicates that

"A tax of $2 per pack of cigarettes can be justified."

smokers cost employers several hundred dollars per year more than nonsmokers. If "how-to-quit" sessions resulted in a high percentage of smokers quitting permanently, the payback period for the employer could be short. The cheapest and most effective measure, however, would be the simple prohibition of smoking in the workplace.[101]

It is ironic that one of the world's most serious epidemics, smoking, is self-inflicted. Some health leaders believe that smoking will eventually become broadly unacceptable. G. Everett Koop, the U.S. Surgeon General, has recently set a goal of a "smoke-free society by the year 2000." By endorsing this goal, political leaders everywhere could promote a profoundly effective but inexpensive public health remedy.

High Technology

Lewis Thomas, Chancellor of the Memorial Sloan-Kettering Cancer Center, argues that technology has been the driving force of modern medicine, and that human health can be improved at an affordable cost only by advancing technology through basic research. Thomas divides health technology into three categories. "High technology" includes vaccines and antibiotics that precisely prevent or cure diseases. They work through detailed understanding, or at least empirical evidence, of underlying mechanisms of cause and effect. Polio vaccine and penicillin exemplify high technology, and diagnostic techniques also belong in this category. The eradication of smallpox is a great triumph of high technology. "Half-way technology," according to Thomas, includes those systems or devices that relieve symptoms, but do not cure disease. The iron lung, which extends the lives of polio victims, is a half-way technology, as is coronary by-pass surgery and many of the treatments for cancer. Thomas' third level is "no technology," about all medicine can offer for nodular melanoma, AIDS, and dozens of other diseases. Recent research, however, has led to a better understanding of AIDS, and, as is the goal of basic research, may soon lead to useful therapies.[102]

Thomas' three categories focus evaluation of medical technology on its purpose, which is to lengthen and improve the quality of human life. Widespread resentment of technology is partly due to the use of new machines and technologies without properly considering their effectiveness and costs. Recent studies of radical mastectomy, for example, illustrate that a medical technology can be used for decades without convincing evidence that it extends life any longer than simpler, less traumatic techniques.[103] Nevertheless, proper immunological, diagnostic, and hospital techniques provide vast benefit for health. Making these tools more widely available and less costly will be part of any successful health strategy.

Inoculations of both antibiotics and preventive serums clearly demonstrate the elegance and cost-effectiveness of high technology as defined by Thomas. Polio cases in the United States dropped from 29,000 per year in 1955, when the vaccine was introduced, to 3,000 only five years later, and to just 8 cases in 1975. Cases are now reported only where people have not been fully immunized. Measles cases dropped by 80 percent after a vaccine was introduced in the sixties.[104] Inoculations that effectively prevent these diseases cost just a few cents each.

Research on similar treatments and cures for tropical and Third World diseases has been neglected, however. The vastly inequitable distribution of wealth in the world is paralleled by a maldistribution of health care research and development. Two-thirds of all resources for health research are spent by the United States, Japan, and Europe, who obviously place lower priority on attacking tropical diseases.[105] Though these maladies afflict over half of mankind, they receive relatively little attention.

Applied research can succeed anywhere that resources are committed to it. The principle on which oral rehydration therapy (ORT) is based had been discovered much earlier in the United States, but had been ignored because no use was seen for it. Researchers working on diarrheal dehydration in Bangladesh rediscovered the principle and used it to develop ORT at a cost of only a few million dollars. Now ORT can be applied for pennies per treatment, though its delivery to several hundred million poor children has yet to be accomplished. Basic research can therefore make major contributions with small commitments of resources.

> "Biotechnology offers great hope for controlling malaria."

A vaccine for malaria would provide the means to relieve the suffering of 300 million people. People free of malaria could do the hard work of development, which malaria impedes perhaps more than any other illness. Scarce food supplies would also be conserved, because a malarial infection requires an additional 2,500 calories per day at the height of illness. Malaria prevention has historically relied on controlling the mosquitos that transmit the organism causing malaria. But mosquitos have developed resistance to pesticides, and the sporozoites have developed resistance to drugs such as chloriquine. The cost of conventional malaria control methods is high, as indicated by the fact that half of India's health budget is allocated to malaria prevention and treatment. Fortunately, biotechnology offers great hope for controlling malaria.[106]

Recombinant DNA and mono-clonal antibodies technologies are being applied by researchers in several Western countries to develop anti-malarial vaccines. The strategy is to develop a compound that would attack the malarial organism, Plasmodium, at a vulnerable stage in its complex life cycle in the human body. By identifying molecules on the surfaces of the cells of the organism at different stages, compounds can be created to neutralize their ability to infect human blood cells, or to prevent their transmission back to a mosquito. Alternatively, vaccines could be devised to destroy infected human blood cells. Recent technical progress has reinforced the belief that a vaccine may be available within a few years. Institutional conflict between research sponsors, including the World Health Organization (WHO) and private drug companies conducting the research, however, has delayed development of this urgently needed medicine. Companies conducting the research wanted to be guaranteed a minimum period of time during which they could exclusively distribute the drug. The WHO wants the patent to be available for any company.[107]

More effective formulas are needed to prevent or cure cholera, schistosomiasis, river blindness, sleeping sickness, parasites, and other tropical diseases. The best vaccine for cholera available today, for example, provides immunity for only about six months and risks producing the very disease it is supposed to prevent because killed viruses are used to provide immunity. Even if only a small fraction survives, the results can be catastrophic. Through genetic engineering, however, scientists may be close to developing an improved cholera vaccine. By reproducing and injecting in the body a particular carbohydrate from the cholera virus cell wall, one that the body's immune system will interpret as the virus itself, immunity can be conferred. More biomedical research such as this is needed, but research costs, though comparatively cheap, are not trivial, and support from governments and foundations has been weak.[108]

Unlike vaccines and antibiotics, half-way technology can be devastatingly expensive. Hospital technologies account for half of the health budgets in developing countries and a third in developed countries. Hospital care now consumes about 3 percent of the entire U.S. Gross National Product. Much of this money is well spent. For those with coronary artery disease, for example, by-pass surgery can mean life, or at least a life worth living and free of pain. Technologies for the treatment of trauma and other high priorities could carry great benefit for developing countries; yet, most developing countries have only one hospital bed for every 600 people, compared to one bed for every 100 people in the developed world.[109] Because their resources are much more limited, developing countries will not soon be able to copy standard practices in developed world hospitals. Doctors will have to learn a variety of common procedures, rather than specialize. The most essential surgery can be identified and given priority.[110]

The Computed Tomography (CT) scanner symbolizes the problem of cost-effectiveness in hospital technology. CT scans provide information similar to X-rays but with far greater detail and with less radiation exposure to the patient. The United States has now installed one of these diagnostic machines, at a cost of about $1 million each, for every 200,000 people. Though CT scanners were invented in the United Kingdom, only one-fourth as many have been installed there on a per capita basis. In the United States, until recently, hospitals or doctors had no incentive to cut costs, while the U.K. government sets specific budgets for medical care. As a result, British doctors are strongly motivated to reduce costly services that benefit relatively few people. Health care there is rationed at a lower level of service. Similar ration-

> "Half-way technology
> can be devastatingly expensive."

ing of Medicare has begun in the United States, with hospitals paid a pre-arranged sum for certain treatments.[111]

Mortality and life span statistics suggest that the British have not suffered from health care rationing, at least compared to Americans. But these figures say little about the comparative quality of life in the two countries. People in the United Kingdom can wait as long as four years for an artificial hip implant. Fewer hip transplants and less heart surgery do mean reduced quality of life for many. But health care in the United States costs twice as much per capita as in the United Kingdom.[112]

The cost of technologies cannot be evaluated apart from their effectiveness. Diagnostic tools such as CT scanners and endoscopes replace more invasive techniques such as surgery and so reduce risk and free hospital beds and surgical teams for other treatments. One study in Norway indicated that CT scanners reduced exploratory surgery by an estimated 90 percent. In developing countries, where hospital facilities are scarce, improved diagnosis can be a good investment.[113]

The high cost of medical technology may be due to consumer demand and the absence of cost-cutting incentives as much as to the capital cost of the technologies themselves. For example, fiber optic endoscopy to probe the remotest locations in the human digestive tract has recently added enormous diagnostic power. The procedure costs only about $45 in the United States, but hospitals charge an average of six to seven times that amount. The difference largely reflects a lack of incentive to avoid the cost—insurance will pay—as well as strong incentives to provide the service.[114]

A flaw in Thomas' categorization is that behavioral science fits poorly or not at all. Society's inability to deal with behavioral disorders is indicated in the costs of homicide, suicide, alcoholism and drug abuse, divorce, smoking, and obesity. Because some disorders such as schizophrenia may be due to chemical imbalances, basic biomedical research could prove very beneficial. It is clear, however, that many problem behaviors—from violent aggression to alcohol abuse—are learned. Overconsumption of alcohol may rival tobacco as a public health problem, and some experts have proposed similar methods to combat it, including banning advertising. Others point out that attaching a social stigma to drinking might discourage drinking in moderation and encourage binge and excessive drinking. Government regulations often usefully change behavior. A law in Australia requiring seatbelts to be worn reduced urban accident mortality by 20 percent. Learning why people smoke and overeat, and how to help them change, will be a much more complex task. Behavioral science, unfortunately, is a vastly underfunded field.[115]

The "technological imperative," the pressure to develop and use new systems no matter how inappropriate, poses a real and growing problem. But misallocating resources for technology development is a greater danger. Improved health care depends on new research and reevaluation of existing knowledge. But biomedical research need not be duplicated all over the world while the most basic tools—stethoscopes, scales, antibiotics, refrigerators, X-ray machines—are absent from developing countries. Financial aid can contribute greatly by providing these tools, the training to use them, and the operating costs of sustaining them.[116]

Both high-and half-way medical technologies offer vast potential for improving the human condition. Balancing their capacity for good against their cost places great stress on human institutions, which must make life-or-death decisions in ways in which they are unaccustomed. The purchase of one expensive machine may mean life for a few and and the denial of resources for life for many others. The capability to keep very premature infants and very ill elderly alive at great expense presents a choice that cannot be made by doctors alone, or even by the families of the victims. Choices between high, half-way, and even no technology are by no means clear cut, and the correct choice will sometimes be to do nothing at all. Making these choices now requires a broader understanding in society of medicine and medical technology.

> "Behavioral science is a vastly underfunded field."

Conclusion

Least-cost health strategies will accord priority to preventive and primary methods designed to attack the world's leading causes of unnecessary death. The toll of childhood infections can be sharply cut by extending primary health care to the world's poor women and children. The cost would total only $10 billion per year—less than two-tenths of a percent of the world's annual economic output—and some five to ten million lives would be saved annually. Where the incidence of diarrheal, tropical, and parasitic diseases are highest, tens of billions of dollars worth of investments in wells and toilets will be necessary, but cost-effective. The toll of heart disease and cancer in middle age can probably be halved with diet modification and the control of smoking. Educational campaigns for reducing fat and cholesterol consumption, coupled with taxes on tobacco and restrictions on public smoking, can help extend millions of lives into old age, and at a favorable cost, compared with the half-way treatments available once the diseases have been acquired. But the best hope of low-cost cures to high-cost diseases such as malaria, sleeping sickness, and the cancers and diseases of the heart not yet understood lies in basic science. Fortunately, the additional cost of research and development would be comparatively low.

These elements of health provision deserve a high priority for public funds and human resources because they will effectively and cheaply save the largest number of lives. They also have a special urgency because their implementation is long overdue.

Emphasizing these five program elements does not diminish the importance of treating other acute ills. Reducing the toll from birth defects, highway accidents, falls, suicide, and homicide remains important. When a health investment such as air bags for reducing automobile fatalities is cost-effective, it can be made profitably, for it will pay for itself both in human and economic terms. Alcohol abuse, at least in the United States, exacts a high human and economic cost, and may not be generally preventable without new developments in behavioral science. Neither economic nor equity policy can justify neglect of these problems simply because their costs are outweighed by greater ones.

But even the largest opportunities for improving the human condition continue to be neglected. Primary health care is tragically underfunded, both in the training of appropriate personnel and in creation of delivery systems. Little funding is provided for appropriate sanitation alternatives. Diet education is haphazard at best, and anti-smoking efforts are sporadic. The policy failure common across these categories is a failure in the field of public health. Government health agencies around the world have been content to foster and develop private, intensive health care, and have allowed preventive and effective primary measures to languish. Preventive medicine comprises less than 2 percent of the training of U.S.-educated doctors.[117]

Governments have an ultimate responsibility for the health and welfare of their people. Many observers believe that sufficient resources exist in developing countries to extend primary health care to all by the year 2000. Recurrent costs will ultimately have to be covered by the beneficiaries of the health services. Fortunately, some curative services can be provided cheaply enough for most to afford. Charging small fees for such services actually enhances their credibility, and the provision of curative services makes the preventive services more acceptable. The initial costs of health-workers training, facilities, equipment, and drugs will almost always have to come from an investment by the governments themselves or through external assistance. Charitable and religious organizations have made large contributions here, but their resources are far too limited to accomplish the task at hand. Governments can reallocate funds to higher priority primary care by saving on wasteful practices in tertiary care systems. Only by reallocating funds from other sectors of their economies, however, can they avoid diminishing the services provided in these centers.

Governments would be more inclined to take action if leaders were judged on their country's state of health. Poverty, inequity, and inefficiency may be covered up in short-run economic statistics, but infant mortality statistics reveal these clearly. Unfortunately, two-thirds of the world is ruled dictatorially, and the leaders thus are not account-

> "Sufficient resources exist to extend primary health care to all."

able to their people. In these nations, pressure must come from the outside. The World Health Organization, the United Nations Childrens' Fund, the International Red Cross, and other world health leaders already serve in this capacity, and their efforts should be strongly supported and extended.

Multilateral and bilateral aid can supplement the health resources of poor nations. Sweden, for example, has long contributed about one percent of its gross economic product for aid, and usually requires that its funds go to the neediest in the promotion of equity and democracy. Aid can contribute best to "investing in people," in their health and education. When children are nourished, mentally sound, and strong, they can better take advantage of the educational opportunities available to them, and help themselves. The developed world as a whole, however, contributes only three-tenths of a percent of its total economic product to development aid. If the richest 20 percent of the world followed Sweden's example, development aid would be tripled, and more than $85 billion would be available each year, part of which could support basic primary health care and sanitation needs. Unfortunately, most aid—even Sweden's—has strings attached. Even if political concessions are not exacted, it usually is required that the beneficiaries spend much of the money buying the products and services of the donor. Such restrictions severely limit the benefit of aid.

In developed countries, the economic benefits of labeling foods, training doctors and teachers in nutrition, and providing dietary education will be enormous, and the costs almost trivial, compared with the alternative.

Tobacco control will require many decisions on many governmental levels. Strong health warnings and the prohibition of advertising are critical first steps. A tax on cigarettes of $2 per pack would discourage smoking and place the burden of smoking's costs to society on the smoker. Restricting public smoking would protect the health of non-smokers. Progress will be painfully slow and difficult in the best of circumstances, and, for this reason, leadership at the highest levels of government will be critical. Parties with vested interests, the medical insurance industry for pecuniary reasons, and the health care industry for ethical reasons, can take the lead in pressuring governments to implement these public health priorities. Citizens and health promotion organizations will need broad support, both financial and political, to be effective.

Closing with a call for more research is a timeworn practice, but one that is justified both by the enormous contribution basic research has made to human health this century and by the equally great potential that biomedical science promises. Recent advances in biotechnology, biochemistry, and genetics may revolutionize medicine around the world. Applying this potential for the good of all humanity, however, is a challenge that may not be met. For along with the maldistribution of wealth goes the maldistribution of science. Rich countries—and their scientists—have an ethical responsibility to allocate a share of this good fortune to solving the problems of the poor.

Notes

1. World Health Organization and United Nations Children's Fund, *Alma-Ata 1978: Primary Health Care: Report of the International Conference on Primary Health Care* (Geneva: World Health Organization, 1978).

2. *The State of the World's Children, 1984* (New York: Oxford University Press, 1983), Statistical Appendix.

3. *Health Sector Policy Paper* (Washington, D.C.: World Bank, 1980).

4. *World Development Report 1983* (New York: Oxford University Press, published for the World Bank, 1983).

5. Income projections assume that growth will not exceed 5.5 percent and that incomes now average less than $400 per capita in half the world. Current income levels were taken from *World Development Report 1983*.

6. The relationship between infant mortality and income was estimated using a simple linear regression analysis with data from *State of the World's Children* (The correlation coefficient (r) equals $-.5$ for countries with incomes less than $1,500 per capita, and $-.4$, between income and infant mortality above 100 per 1,000).

7. David Banta, deputy director of the Pan American Health Organization, Washington, D.C., private communication, February 1, 1984; Hector R. Acuna, *Toward 2000: The Quest for Universal Health in the Americas* (Washington, D.C.: Pan American Health Organization, 1983); *Health Conditions in the Americas 1977-1980* (Washington, D.C.: Pan American Health Organization, 1982); *State of the World's Children*.

8. *State of the World's Children*; and Pedro N. Acha and Boris Szyfres, *Zoonoses and Communicable Diseases Common to Man and Animals* (Washington, D.C.: Pan American Health Organization, 1981).

9. World Bank, Poverty and Basic Needs Series, "Water Supply and Waste Disposal," Washington, D.C., 1983; *Health Sector Policy Paper*; "Mortality and Health Policy: Highlights of the Issues in the Context of the World Population Plan of Action," draft report of the Population Division of the Department of International Economic and Social Affairs, United Nations, New York, May 4, 1983.

10. National Center for Health Statistics, *Health: United States, 1982* (Washington, D.C.: U.S. Government Printing Office, 1982); *State of the World's Children*.

11. *Health Conditions in the Americas 1977-1980*.

12. *State of the World's Children*; B. N. Ames, "Dietary Carcinogens and Anticarcinogens," *Science*, September 23, 1983; James B. Wyngaarden and Lloyd H. Smith, Jr., eds., *Cecil Textbook of Medicine* (Philadelphia: W.B. Saunders Company, 1982); Derek Bok, "Needed: A New Way to Train Doctors," *Harvard Magazine*, May-June, 1984; Richard Doll and Richard Peto, "Quantitative Estimates of Avoidable Risks of Cancer in the United States Today, *Journal of the National Cancer Institute*, November 1981.

13. Patricia W. Blair, ed., *Health Needs of the World's Poor Women* (Washington, D.C.: Equity Policy Center, 1981).

14. David Banta, private communication, February 1, 1984.

15. *State of the World's Children*.

16. *Cecil Textbook of Medicine*.

17. Daniel Yohalem, "American Children in Poverty," Children's Defense Fund, Washington, D.C., 1984; *State of the World's Children*.

18. John R. Evans, Karen Lashman Hall, and Jeremy Warford, "Health Care in the Developing World: Problems of Scarcity and Choice," *The New England Journal of Medicine*, November 5, 1981; Margaret Burns Parlato, *Primary Health Care: An Analysis of 52 AID-Assisted Projects* (Washington, D.C.: American Public Health Association, 1982); Rashid Faruqee, "Analysing the Impact of Health Services, Project Experience from India, Ghana, and Thailand," World Bank Staff Working Papers, Number 546, Washington, D.C., 1982; *State of the World's Children; Health Sector Policy Paper*.

19. W. Henry Mosley, "Will Primary Health Care Reduce Infant and Child Mortality? A Critique of Some Current Strategies, with Special Reference to Africa and Asia," draft report of the Ford Foundation to the United Nations Conference on Population.

20. *State of the World's Children*.

21. R. G. Whitehead, ed., *Maternal Diet, Breast-feeding Capacity, and Lactational Infertility* (Tokyo: The United Nations University, 1983).

22. "Findings of the World Fertility Survey on Trends, Differentials and Determinants of Mortality in Developing Countries," prepared by the Secretariat of the World Fertility Survey for the 1984 International Conference on Population, May 3, 1983.

23. Kathleen Newland, *Infant Mortality and the Health of Societies*, (Washington, D.C.: Worldwatch Institute, 1981); Galba Araujo et al. "Improving Obstetric Care In Northeast Brazil," *Bulletin of the Pan American Health Organization*, Volume 17, No. 3, 1983.

24. *Health Conditions in the Americas; State of the World's Children*.

25. *Cecil Textbook of Medicine*.

26. *Health Sector Policy Paper*; David Banta, private communication; James Heiby, Deputy Director, Health Services Division, U.S. Agency for International Development, private communication, June 8, 1984; *State of the World's Children*.

27. Lester R. Brown, *Building A Sustainable Society* (New York: W.W. Norton, & Co., 1981); *State of the World's Children; Health Sector Policy Paper*; "Findings of the World Fertility Survey on Trends, Differentials, and Determinants of Mortality in Developing Countries."

28. *Maternal Diet, Breast-feeding Capacity, and Lactational Infertility*; Lloyd Harbert and Pasquale L. Scandizzo, "Food Distribution and Nutrition Intervention: The Case of Chile," World Bank Working Papers, Number 512, Washington, D.C., May 1982; Pasquale L. Scandizzo, and Gurushri Swamy, "Benefits and Costs of Food Distribution Policies: The India Case," World Bank Working Papers, Number 509, Washington, D.C., 1982.

29. S. N. Tibrewala and K. P. Shah, "The Use of Arm Circumference as an Indicator of Body Weight in Adult Women," *Baroda Journal of Nutrition*, Vol. 5, No. 43, 1978, as cited in World Federation of Public Health Associations, "Maternal Nutrition: Information for Action Resource Guide," Washington, D.C., July 1983.

30. "Infant and Child Mortality in Rural Areas: Implications for Rural Development Programmes," prepared by the Food and Agriculture Organization of the United Nations for the 1984 International Conference on Population, May 3, 1983; R. V. Short, "Breast Feeding," *Scientific American*, April 1984; *State of the World's Children; Maternal Diet, Breast-feeding Capacity, and Lactational Infertility*.

31. F. C. Ramsey, "An Analysis of Breast-Feeding Findings in the Barbados National Health and Nutrition Surveys of 1969 and 1981, With Special Reference to the International Code of Marketing of Breast-milk Substitutes," *CAJANUS* 16(1):14-18, 1983, as cited in *Bulletin of the Pan American Health Organization*, Volume 17, No. 3, 1983.

32. *Cecil Textbook of Medicine.*

33. *Cecil Textbook of Medicine* and *State of the World's Children.*

34. *State of the World's Children.*

35. Rashid Faruqee and Ethna Johnson, "Health, Nutrition, and Family Planning in India: A Survey of Experiments and Special Projects," World Bank Working Papers, Number 507, Washington, D.C., February 1982. For descriptions of the Chinese primary care system, see Ruth Sidel, *Women and Child Care in China* (Baltimore: Penguin Books, 1974) and Wu Naitao, "The Healthy Growth of China's Children," *Beijing Review,* June 25, 1984.

36. "Modern Medicine is Quickly Gaining Acceptance," *New York Times,* December 28, 1983.

37. "Health, Nutrition, and Family Planning in India."

38. *Ibid.*

39. Warren L. Berggren, Douglas C. Ewbank, and Gretchen G. Berggren, "Reduction of Mortality in Rural Haiti Through A Primary-Health-Care Program," the *New England Journal of Medicine,* May 28, 1981.

40. "Health, Nutrition, and Family Planning In India."

41. "Primary Health Care: Progress and Problems, An Analysis of 52 AID-assisted Projects"; "Reduction of Mortality in Rural Haiti Through A Primary-Health-Care Program"; "Health, Nutrition, and Family Planning In India"; George Alleyne, director, Regional Programs Development, Pan American Health Organization, private communication, April 10, 1984.

42. Yusif Ali Fraj, "Point of View: No One Is Realistic About Family Planning," *World Health Forum,* Volume 4, No. 2 1983.

43. *Alma-Ata 1978: Primary Health Care.*

44. *World Military and Social Expenditures, 1983; Health Sector Policy Paper; State of the World's Children.*

45. *IDA In Retrospect: The First Two Decades of the International Development Association* (New York: Oxford University Press, 1982); *Security and Development Assistance,* Hearings before the Committee On Foreign Relations, United States Senate, February through March, 1983 (Washington, D.C.: U.S. Government Printing Office, 1983); *World Development Report 1983.*

46. *Toward 2000: The Quest for Universal Health in the Americas*; David Banta, private communication; George Alleyne, private communication.

47. *Amnesty International Report, 1983* (London: Amnesty International Publications, 1983).

48. Peter Bourne, president, Global Water, Inc., private communication, April 3, 1984.

49. *Safe Water and Waste Disposal for Rural Health*; *Health Conditions in the Americas*; *Health Sector Policy Paper*; "Water Supply and Waste Disposal."

50. John M. Hunter, Luis Rey, and David Scott, "Man-made Lakes—Man-made Diseases," *World Health Forum*, Vol. 3, No. 2, 1983; Paul L. Aspelin and Silvio Coelho das Santos, *Indian Areas Threatened By Hydro-electric Projects in Brazil* (Copenhagen: International Working Group for Indigenous Affairs, 1981); *Safe Water and Waste Disposal For Rural Health*.

51. John M. Kalbermatten et al., *Appropriate Sanitation Alternatives* (Baltimore: The Johns Hopkins University Press, 1982).

52. Charles E. Rosenberg, *The Cholera Years: The United States in 1832, 1849, and 1866* (Chicago: The University of Chicago Press, 1962); *Health Sector Policy Paper*; Department of Rural Water Supply, National Sanitary Works, Chile, "Drinking Water: A Determinant of Health," *World Health Forum*, Volume 4, No. 2, 1983.

53. Edmond de Gaiffier and Michel Jancloes, "Financial Analysis: A Critical Determinant For the Viability of Health Programmes," draft report prepared for the 1984 International Conference on Population; *Health Sector Policy Paper*.

54. Sumi Krishna Chauhan, "Water a Necessity, Clean Water a Luxury," *Pakistan and Gulf Economist*, November 19-25, 1983.

55. "Will Primary Health Care Reduce Infant and Child Mortality? A Critique of Some Current Strategies, With Special Reference to Africa and Asia."

56. Peter Bourne, private communication, April 9, 1984; *Safe Water and Waste Disposal*; "The Myths of the Water Decade," *Ecoforum*, Vol. 8, No. 6, 1983; *Village Water Supply*; F. Eugene McJunkin, "Water and Human Health, National Water Demonstration Project, prepared for the U.S. Agency for International Development, Washington, D.C., July, 1982.

57. Peter Bourne, private communication.

58. *Village Water Supply*; "Water Supply and Waste Disposal."

59. *Appropriate Sanitation Alternatives.*

60. *Human Waste Management For Low-Income Settlements* (Bangkok: Environmental Sanitation Information Center, 1983); Peter Bourne, private communication.

61. *Human Waste Management*; Bindeshwar Pathak, *Sulabh Shauchalaya: Hand Flush Water Seal Latrine, A Simple Idea That Worked* (Calcutta: Amola Prakashan, Patna, 1981).

62. *Sulabh Shauchalaya: Hand Flush Water Seal Latrine; Sulabh Shauchalaya: A Study of Directed Change* (New Delhi: Amola Press and Publications, 1982).

63. *Human Waste Management; Appropriate Sanitation Alternatives.*

64. William U. Chandler, *The Myth of TVA: Conservation and Development in the Tennessee Valley, 1933-1983* (Cambridge, Mass.: Ballinger Publishing Company, 1984).

65. Colin Glennie, "A Model for the Development of a Self-help Water Supply Program," World Bank Technical Paper Number 2, Washington, D.C., 1982.

66. For further development of this theme, see Theodore W. Schultz, *Investing in People: The Economics of Population Quality* (Berkeley, Calif.: University of California Press, 1981).

67. "The Causes of Cancer: Quantitative Estimates of Avoidable Risks of Cancer in the United States Today"; "Dietary Carcinogens and Anticarcinogens, *"Diet, Nutrition, and Cancer* (Washington, D.C.: National Academy Press, 1982); Antonio M. Gotto, Jr., "Statement About Results of Coronary Prevention Trial," news release of the American Heart Association, Washington, D.C., January 10, 1984; Lipid Research Clinics Program, "The Lipid Research Clinics Coronary Primary Prevention Trial Results: Reduction in Incidence of Coronary Heart Disease," *Journal of the American Medical Association*, January 20, 1984; Michael Gough et al., U.S. Congress Office of Technology Assessment, *Assessment of Technologies for Determining Cancer Risks From the Environment* (Washington, D.C.: U.S. Government Printing Office, June 1981); "Prevention Pays Off," press release of the National Cancer Institute announcing the initiation of a cancer prevention campaign, March 6, 1984. But for opposing views, see, "Letters: Cancer and Diet," *Science*, May 18, 1984; John R. Totter, "Spontaneous Cancer and Its Possible Relationship to Oxygen Metabolism," *Proceedings of the National Academy of Sciences, USA*,

April 1980; Council for Agricultural Science and Technology, "Diet, Nutrition, and Cancer: A Critique," Ames, Iowa, October, 1982.

68. "The Causes of Cancer: Quantitative Estimates of Avoidable Risks of Cancer in the United States Today"; *Diet, Nutrition, and Cancer; World Health Statistics Annual, 1982* (Geneva: World Health Organization, 1982).

69. Lipid Research Clinics Program, "The Lipid Research Clinics Coronary Primary Prevention Trial Results: The Relationship of Reduction in Incidence of Coronary Heart Disease to Cholesterol Lowering," *Journal of the American Medical Association*, January 20, 1984.

70. *Cecil Textbook of Medicine*; Lubert Stryer, *Biochemistry* (San Francisco: W.H. Freeman and Company, 1981).

71. *Cecil Textbook of Medicine*; "The Lipid Research Clinics Coronary Primary Prevention Trial Results: Reduction in Incidence of Coronary Heart Disease."

72. John Lagona, "Heart Attack and Cholesterol," *Discover*, March 1984.

73. *Cecil Textbook of Medicine; Diet, Nutrition, and Cancer.*

74. Derived from *Health: United States 1982*, and *Assessment of Technologies For Determining Cancer Risks From The Environment*.

75. Liane Russell, Section Head, Mammalian Genetics Section, Oak Ridge National Laboratory, private communication, June 6, 1984.

76. *Diet, Nutrition, and Cancer*; National Cancer Institute press release; Jane E. Brody, *Jane Brody's Nutrition Book* (New York: W.W. Norton, & Co., 1981).

77. Worldwatch Institute analysis of foodstuffs as described in U.S. Department of Agriculture, "Nutritive Value of Foods," Washington, D.C., revised, April 1981 and in *Jane Brody's Nutrition Book*.

78. Ruth M. Marston and Susan O. Welsh, "Nutrient Content of the U.S. Food Supply, 1982," *National Food Review*, Winter 1984.

79. *Health: United States, 1982; Cecil Textbook of Medicine.*

80. For an assessment of the literature on the benefits and costs of preventive medicine, see, Louise Russell, "The Economics of Prevention," Brookings Institution, February 1984, unpublished version of a paper presented at the 1982 Frank M. Norfleet Forum for the Advancement of Health, University of

Tennessee Center for the Health Services, Memphis, Tennessee. See also, Shan Cretin, "Cost/Benefit Analysis of Treatment and Prevention of Myocardial Infarction," *Health Services Research*, Summer 1977; Kenneth E. Warner and Rebecca C. Hutton, "Cost-Benefit and Cost-Effectiveness Analysis in Health Care," *Medical Care*, November 1980; and Jeffrey P. Koplan et al., "Pertussis Vaccine—An Analysis of Benefits, Risks, and Costs, The *New England Journal of Medicine*, October 25, 1979; for a survey of preventive programs, see, Office of Cancer Communications, "Planning A Cancer Prevention Program: Review of Health and Prevention Campaigns," National Cancer Institute, undated mimeo.

81. *Cecil Textbook of Medicine; Health: United States, 1982*; Phillip M. Boffey, "U.S. Reports Gains in Nation's Health," *New York Times*, January 1, 1984; *Levels and Trends of Mortality Since 1950* (New York: United Nations, 1982); "Nutrient Content of the U.S. Food Supply, 1982"; John Weisburger, director, Naylor Dana Institute For Disease Prevention, private communication, June 21, 1984.

82. Rose Mary Romano, Chief, Information Projects Branch, Office of Cancer Communications, National Cancer Institute, private communication, June 19, 1984; see also, Office of Cancer Communications, "Cancer Prevention Research Summary—Nutrition," National Cancer Institute, February 1984; *Statistical Abstracts of the United States* (Washington, D.C.: U.S. Government Printing Office, 1983).

83. These illustrative labels were derived as follows. For cholesterol, maximum dietary intakes of 300 and 225 milligrams per day for men and women, respectively, were assumed, as recommended by the American Heart Association. (See American Heart Association, "Recommendations for Treatment of Hyperlipidemia In Adults," Dallas, Texas, 1983). For fat, the maximum dietary consumption of 30 percent of daily calorie consumption was assumed, as recommended by the National Cancer Institute. (See press statement of Health and Human Services Secretary Margaret Heckler, "Cancer Prevention Awareness Program Press Conference," March 6, 1984 and Rose Mary Romano, private communication.) Calorie RDAs were assumed to be 2,700 and 2,100 for males and females, respectively. (See National Academy of Sciences—National Research Council, "Recommended Dietary Allowances," 1980.) The cholesterol and fat composition of foods were obtained from U.S. Department of Agriculture, "Nutritive Value of Foods," Washington, D.C., April 1981, and U.S.D.A. data as cited in *Jane Brody's Nutrition Book*.

84. Michael Jacobson, executive director, Center for Science in the Public Interest, private communication, June 21, 1983.

85. Gerry Oster, Graham A. Colditz, Nancy L. Kelly, *The Economic Costs of Smoking and Benefits of Quitting* (Lexington, Mass.: Lexington Books, 1984).

86. The average discount rate applied in these studies was 5 percent. See "The Economics of Prevention."

87. David Banta, private communication; Clyde Behney, private communication, June 18, 1984.

88. This claim can be illustrated by using the detailed estimates of the lifetime costs of death due to coronary heart disease made by Oster et al., in *The Economic Costs of Smoking and Benefits of Quitting*, which, at age 55, amount to more than $200,000, discounted to onset of the disease. Then, assuming that only half the population of the U.S. dies of heart disease, that 25 percent of all heart disease victims die before age 65, that only half these cases could be avoided, and that an intervention program would be effective in only 10 percent of these cases, the net present value of such a program per case avoided would be around $1,250. Thus, a $50 screening program applied at age 35 and discounted at 3 percent would have a net present cost of less than $100, less than one-twelfth the total benefits. Alternatively, such a screening program could be applied twelve times and would break even in costs and benefits, and would more than break even if the reduced costs of morbidity were added, or if it were assumed that the effectiveness of preventive measures increased with the number of interventions.

89. *Cecil Textbook of Medicine*; David Banta, private communication; *Diet, Nutrition, and Cancer*; "The Causes of Cancer: Quantitative Estimates of Avoidable Risks of Cancer in the United States Today"; *Health: United States, 1982;* Royal College of Physicians of London, *Smoking or Health*, (London: Pitman Publishing Ltd, 1983); Dorothy P. Rice and Thomas A. Hodgson, "Economic Costs of Smoking: An Analysis of Data for the United States," draft report presented at the Allied Social Science Association Annual Meetings, San Francisco, California, December 28, 1983; Bryan R. Luce and Stuart O. Schweitzer, "Smoking and Alcohol Abuse: A Comparison of their Economic Consequences," *New England Journal of Medicine*, March 9, 1978; Worldwatch estimates of expenditures on cigarettes.

90. Stuart Jay Olshansky, "Is Smoker/Nonsmoker Segregation Effective in Reducing Passive Inhalation Among Nonsmokers?" *American Journal of Public Health*, July 1982; *Cecil Textbook of Medicine*. Note that the reference to carbon monoxide content of the blood technically means the percent of blood composed of carboxyhemoglobin.

91. *Cecil Textbook of Medicine; Diet, Nutrition, and Cancer;* "The Causes of Cancer: Quantitative Estimates of Avoidable Risks of Cancer in the United States Today"; *Health: United States, 1982;* "Smoking and Health," *Report of the Surgeon General,* U.S. Department of Health, Education, and Welfare, Washington, D.C., 1979.

92. *Smoking or Health; Report of the Advisory Committee to the Surgeon General of the U.S. Public Health Service,* January 11, 1984; "Fact Sheet: Trends in Cigarette Consumption, 1964-1984," Office on Smoking and Health, U.S. Public Health Service, January, 1984.; Nicholas Cohen, "Smoking and Survival Prospects in Bangledesh," *World Health Forum,* Vol. 3, No. 4, 1982.

93. Kenneth E. Warner and Hillary A. Murt, "Premature Deaths Avoided by the Antismoking Campaign," *American Journal of Public Health,* June 1983; Kenneth E. Warner, "Cigarette Smoking in the 1970's: The Impact of the Antismoking Campaign On Consumption," *Science,* February 13, 1981.

94. Matthew L. Myers et al., "Staff Report on the Cigarette Advertising Investigation," U.S. Federal Trade Commission, May, 1981; *Smoking or Health.*

95. *Statistical Abstracts of the United States, 1982-3* (Washington, D.C.: U.S. Government Printing Office, 1982).

96. For a general description of cigarette advertising in the United States, see Ken Cummins, "The Cigarette Makers: How They Get Away With Murder. . . . With the Press as an Accessory," *The Washington Monthly,* April 1984.

97. *Smoking or Health; ASH: Smoking and Health Review,* May 1984. For a detailed analysis of economic costs of smoking (per individual) see *The Economic Costs of Smoking and Benefits of Quitting;* and "Economic Costs of Smoking: An Analysis of Data for the United States." The U.S. tax rate assumes the tax per pack reverts from 16¢ to 8¢ in 1985, and that the average state tax is just over 15¢ (unweighted). See Tobacco Institute, "Cigarette Tax Data," Washington, D.C., May 14, 1984.

98. "Tariff and Nontariff Measures on Tobacco," Foreign Agriculture Circular, U.S. Department of Agriculture, January 1984; Shim Jae Hoon, "Smoking Can Kill a Career," *Far Eastern Economic Review,* March 1, 1984.

99. Pelayo Correa et al., "Passive Smoking and Lung Cancer," *Lancet,* September 10, 1983; Colin Feyerabend, Tim Higenbottam, and M.A.H. Russell, "Nicotine Concentrations in Urine and Saliva of Smokers and Non-Smokers," *British Medical Journal,* April 3, 1982; Ira B. Tager et al., "Longitudinal Study of the Effects of Maternal Smoking on Pulmonary Function in Children," *The*

New England Journal of Medicine, September 22, 1983; Takeshi Hirayama, "Non-smoking wives of heavy smokers have a higher risk of lung cancer: A Study from Japan," *British Medical Journal*, January 17, 1981; "Is Smoker/Non-Smoker Segregation Effective in Reducing Passive Inhalation Among Non-Smokers?"

100. Judith Cummings, "Restrictions on Smoking Spreading Across U.S.," *New York Times*, March 1, 1984; Judith Cummings, "San Franciscans Adjust to City Curb on Smoking," *New York Times*, March 2, 1984; Jay Mathews, "Stringent Anti-Smoking Law Goes Into Effect in San Francisco," *Washington Post*, March 2, 1984; John Burgess, "Alexandria Tackles Law to Ban Smoking in Most Public Places," *Washington Post*, March 16, 1984; "Alexandria Bans Public Smoking," *Washington Post*, March 18, 1984; Charles Fishman, "Fairfax Prohibits Hiring of Smokers in Safety Jobs," *Washington Post*, March 13, 1984.

101. Preliminary estimate based on work in progress at Policy Analysis, Inc., sponsored by the U.S. Department of Health and Human Services. Gerry Oster, senior economist, Policy Anylysis, Inc., Brookline, Massachusetts, private communication, June 20, 1984.

102. Lewis Thomas, *The Youngest Science* (New York: Viking Press, 1983); Lewis Thomas, "Scientific Frontiers and National Frontiers," *Foreign Affairs*, Spring 1984.

103. Karen Schacter and Duncan Neuhauser, U.S. Congress Office of Technology Assessment, "The Implications of Cost-Effectiveness Analysis of Medical Technology: Case Study #17: Surgery for Breast Cancer," Washington, D.C., U.S. Government Printing Office, October 1981.

104. *Health: United States, 1982.*

105. U.S. Congressional Budget Office, "Federal Support for R & D and Innovation," U.S. Government Printing Office, Washington, D.C., April 1984.

106. D. J. Wyler, "Malaria—Resurgence, Resistance, and Research," *The New England Journal of Medicine*, 1983; U.S. Congress Office of Technology Assessment, *Commercial Biotechnolgy: An International Analysis* (Washington, D.C.: U.S. Government Printing Office, January 1984); "Scientific Frontiers and National Frontiers."

107. W. H. Wernsdorfer, "Prospects for the Development of Malaria Vaccines," *Bulletin of the World Health Organization*, Vol. 59, No. 3, 1981; and *Commercial Biotechnolgy: An International Analysis*.

108. "Reports from Africa: Yellow Fever, Oral Cholera Vaccines," *International Health Magazine*, February-March, 1984. Clyde J. Behney et al., U.S. Congress Office of Technology Assessment, "Quality and Relevance of Research and Related Activities at the Gorgas Memorial Laboratory," U.S. Government Printing Office, Washington, D.C. August 1983; *Security and Development Assistance*.

109. "World Military and Social Expenditures, 1983."

110. George Alleyne, private communication.

111. Henry J. Aaron and William B. Schwartz, *The Painful Prescription: Rationing Hospital Care* (Washington, D.C.: The Brookings Institution, 1984).

112. *The Painful Prescription*.

113. David Banta, private communication; George Alleyne, private communication; Karen Kohlhof et al., U.S. Congress Office of Technology Assessment, *Policy Implications of the Computed Tomography (CT) Scanner: An Update* (Washington, D.C.: U.S. Government Printing Office, January 1981).

114. Clyde J. Behney et al., U.S. Congress Office of Technology Assessment, "Diagnosis Related Groups (DRGs) and the Medicare Program: Implications for Medical Technology," U.S. Government Printing Office, Washington, D.C., July 1983; *The Painful Prescription*; Jonathan A. Showstack and Steven A. Schroeder, U.S. Congress Office of Technology Assessment, "The Implications of Cost-Effectiveness Analysis of Medical Technology, Case Study #8: The Cost Effectiveness of Upper Gastrointestinal Endoscopy," U.S. Government Printing Office, Washington, D.C., May 1981; Clyde Behney, private communication.

115. *Cecil Textbook of Medicine*; Sarnoff A. Mednick, *Learning* (Englewood Cliffs, New Jersey: Prentice-Hall, Inc., 1964; U.S. Congress Office of Technology Assessment, "Mandatory Passive Restraint Systems in Automobile: Issues and Evidence," Washington, D.C., U.S. Government Printing Office, September, 1982; Michael Jacobson, *Nutrition Action*, May, 1984.

116. George Alleyne, private communication.

117. "Needed: A New Way to Train Doctors."

WILLIAM U. CHANDLER is a Senior Researcher at Worldwatch Institute in Washington, D.C. He is co-author of *State of the World 1984, Energy: The Conservation Revolution*, and author of *The Myth of TVA*, as well as many articles on energy and the environment.

THE WORLDWATCH PAPER SERIES

No. of
Copies

1. **The Other Energy Crisis: Firewood** by Erik Eckholm.
2. **The Politics and Responsibility of the North American Breadbasket** by Lester R. Brown.
3. **Women in Politics: A Global Review** by Kathleen Newland.
4. **Energy: The Case for Conservation** by Denis Hayes.
5. **Twenty-two Dimensions of the Population Problem** by Lester R. Brown, Patricia L. McGrath, and Bruce Stokes.
6. **Nuclear Power: The Fifth Horseman** by Denis Hayes.
7. **The Unfinished Assignment: Equal Education for Women** by Patricia L. McGrath.
8. **World Population Trends: Signs of Hope, Signs of Stress** by Lester R. Brown.
9. **The Two Faces of Malnutrition** by Erik Eckholm and Frank Record.
10. **Health: The Family Planning Factor** by Erik Eckholm and Kathleen Newland.
11. **Energy: The Solar Prospect** by Denis Hayes.
12. **Filling The Family Planning Gap** by Bruce Stokes.
13. **Spreading Deserts—The Hand of Man** by Erik Eckholm and Lester R. Brown.
14. **Redefining National Security** by Lester R. Brown.
15. **Energy for Development: Third World Options** by Denis Hayes.
16. **Women and Population Growth: Choice Beyond Childbearing** by Kathleen Newland.
17. **Local Responses to Global Problems: A Key to Meeting Basic Human Needs** by Bruce Stokes.
18. **Cutting Tobacco's Toll** by Erik Eckholm.
19. **The Solar Energy Timetable** by Denis Hayes.
20. **The Global Economic Prospect: New Sources of Economic Stress** by Lester R. Brown.
21. **Soft Technologies, Hard Choices** by Colin Norman.
22. **Disappearing Species: The Social Challenge** by Erik Eckholm.
23. **Repairs, Reuse, Recycling—First Steps Toward a Sustainable Society** by Denis Hayes.
24. **The Worldwide Loss of Cropland** by Lester R. Brown.
25. **Worker Participation—Productivity and the Quality of Work Life** by Bruce Stokes.
26. **Planting for the Future: Forestry for Human Needs** by Erik Eckholm.
27. **Pollution: The Neglected Dimensions** by Denis Hayes.
28. **Global Employment and Economic Justice: The Policy Challenge** by Kathleen Newland.
29. **Resource Trends and Population Policy: A Time for Reassessment** by Lester R. Brown.
30. **The Dispossessed of the Earth: Land Reform and Sustainable Development** by Erik Eckholm.
31. **Knowledge and Power: The Global Research and Development Budget** by Colin Norman.
32. **The Future of the Automobile in an Oil-Short World** by Lester R. Brown, Christopher Flavin, and Colin Norman.
33. **International Migration: The Search for Work** by Kathleen Newland.
34. **Inflation: The Rising Cost of Living on a Small Planet** by Robert Fuller.
35. **Food or Fuel: New Competition for the World's Cropland** by Lester R. Brown.
36. **The Future of Synthetic Materials: The Petroleum Connection** by Christopher Flavin.
37. **Women, Men, and The Division of Labor** by Kathleen Newland.

| | 38. **City Limits: Emerging Constraints on Urban Growth** by Kathleen Newland.
| ___ | 39. **Microelectronics at Work: Productivity and Jobs in the World Economy** by Colin Norman.
| ___ | 40. **Energy and Architecture: The Solar and Conservation Potential** by Christopher Flavin.
| ___ | 41. **Men and Family Planning** by Bruce Stokes.
| ___ | 42. **Wood: An Ancient Fuel with a New Future** by Nigel Smith.
| ___ | 43. **Refugees: The New International Politics of Displacement** by Kathleen Newland.
| ___ | 44. **Rivers of Energy: The Hydropower Potential** by Daniel Deudney.
| ___ | 45. **Wind Power: A Turning Point** by Christopher Flavin.
| ___ | 46. **Global Housing Prospects: The Resource Constraints** by Bruce Stokes.
| ___ | 47. **Infant Mortality and the Health of Societies** by Kathleen Newland.
| ___ | 48. **Six Steps to a Sustainable Society** by Lester R. Brown and Pamela Shaw.
| ___ | 49. **Productivity: The New Economic Context** by Kathleen Newland.
| ___ | 50. **Space: The High Frontier in Perspective** by Daniel Deudney.
| ___ | 51. **U.S. and Soviet Agriculture: The Shifting Balance of Power** by Lester R. Brown.
| ___ | 52. **Electricity from Sunlight: The Future of Photovoltaics** by Christopher Flavin.
| ___ | 53. **Population Policies for a New Economic Era** by Lester R. Brown.
| ___ | 54. **Promoting Population Stabilization: Incentives for Small Families** by Judith Jacobsen
| ___ | 55. **Whole Earth Security: A Geopolitics of Peace** by Daniel Deudney
| ___ | 56. **Materials Recycling: The Virtue of Necessity** by William U. Chandler
| ___ | 57. **Nuclear Power: The Market Test** by Christopher Flavin
| ___ | 58. **Air Pollution, Acid Rain, and the Future of Forests** by Sandra Postel
| ___ | 59. **Improving World Health: A Least Cost Strategy** by William U. Chandler

___ **Total Copies**

Single Copy—$4.00

Bulk Copies (any combination of titles)
    2-5: $3.00 each   5-20: $2.00 each   21 or more: $1.00 each

Calendar Year Subscription (1984 subscription begins with Paper 58)
    U.S. $25.00 ___

Make check payable to Worldwatch Institute
1776 Massachusetts Avenue NW, Washington, D.C. 20036 USA

Enclosed is my check for U.S. $ ___

name

address

city   **state**   **zip/country**

four dollars

Worldwatch Institute
1776 Massachusetts Avenue, N.W.
Washington, D.C. 20036 USA